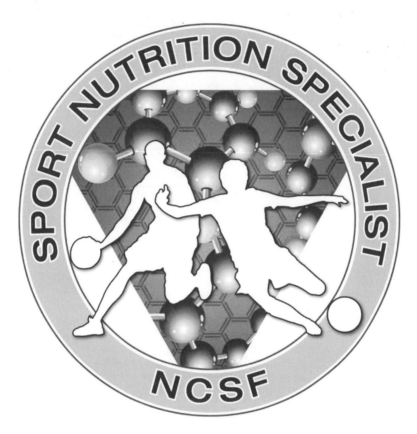

SPORT NUTRITION SPECIALIST

NCSF

National Council on Strength & Fitness

Printed in the United States of America

Library of Congress Control Number: 2007925963

ISBN 978-0-9791696-8-7

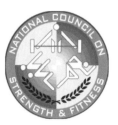

Table of Contents

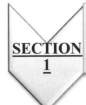

• LEARNING GOALS

Upon completing this section, along with its corresponding chapter, you should understand the following:

1. The relevance and differences between basic nutrition and sport nutrition

2. The different categories and functions of nutrients

3. The key functions, recommended intakes and varying types of carbohydrates

4. The functions and recommended intake of soluble and insoluble fiber

5. Types of lipids and their key functions

6. The functions and structures of varying types of fatty acids

7. Cholesterol and its functions

8. The structure, functions, and recommended intakes for protein

9. The differences between complete and incomplete proteins and their sources

10. The relevance of proper hydration as well as the consequences of dehydration

11. Key functions of fat-soluble and water-soluble vitamins

12. The mechanisms by which phytonutrients may promote enhanced health

SECTION 2 • **QUICKFACTS**

WHAT IS NUTRITION?

- **Nutrition** – total processes of ingestion, digestion, absorption, and metabolism of food
- **Nutrient** – substance in food that performs one or more essential functions in the body
- **Sports Nutrition** – nutrient needs based on specific physiological demands of a given sport
  - Often different than general population needs

Learn More: Sport Nutrition Textbook pg. 2

NUTRITION VS SPORT NUTRITION

- Healthy nutrition guidelines are applicable for all populations but variances can apply

Sedentary Individual
- Total caloric need may be lower
- Lower carbohydrate/high fiber to lower disease risk
- Low sodium to lower disease risk
- Dietary protein need relatively low

Competitive Athlete
- Total caloric need may be higher
- Higher carbohydrate intake based on activity
- Greater sodium for training in heat/humidity
- Dietary protein need higher for strength training

Learn More: Sport Nutrition Textbook pg. 2

CATEGORIES OF NUTRIENTS

- **Macronutrients:** present in the diet in relatively large quantities (>1 g/day)
- **Micronutrients:** present in the diet in small quantities (<1 g/day)

Macronutrients

Carbohydrate
Fat
Protein
Water

Micronutrients

Vitamins
Minerals
Trace Elements

Learn More: Sport Nutrition Textbook pgs. 2-3

FUNCTIONS OF NUTRIENTS

Promotion of growth and development	•Protein – soft tissues, organs, muscles •Minerals – bones, various structures (i.e., calcium, phosphorus)
Provision of energy	•Carbohydrates and fats primary, protein minimal
Regulation of metabolism	•Vitamins, minerals, and proteins (in the form of enzymes)

Learn More: Sport Nutrition Textbook pg. 2

CARBOHYDRATES

- Provide energy for physical activity and exercise performance
  - o Predominant fuel during high-intensity training
  - o Glucose is the only fuel used by the brain and nervous system under normal conditions
- Recommended 45%-65% of the diet depending on activity level and body size
  - o Contrary to recommendations for optimal health, the current Western diet consists of approximately 40-50% carbohydrates with half of the total carbohydrate intake in the form of sugars such as sucrose and high-fructose corn syrups
  - o Yearly sugar intake equates to 50 kg/year (110 lb/year) – 25x more than 100 years ago

Learn More: Sport Nutrition Textbook pgs. 6-8

CLASSES OF CARBOHYDRATES

Monosaccharides Basic unit of carbohydrates (simple sugars)	• Glucose, fructose, galactose
Disaccharides Considered simple sugars	• Sucrose, lactose, maltose (provides 20-25% of energy in Western diet)
Oligosaccharides 3 to 9 monosaccharides combined	• Found in many vegetables
Polysaccharides 10 or more monosaccharides combined	• Starch, glycogen, fiber

Learn More: Sport Nutrition Textbook pgs. 3-5

TYPES OF DIETARY CARBOHYDRATES

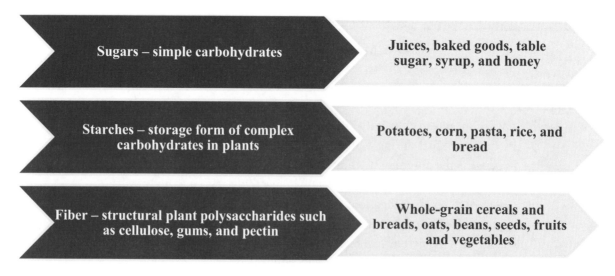

Sugars – simple carbohydrates	Juices, baked goods, table sugar, syrup, and honey
Starches – storage form of complex carbohydrates in plants	Potatoes, corn, pasta, rice, and bread
Fiber – structural plant polysaccharides such as cellulose, gums, and pectin	Whole-grain cereals and breads, oats, beans, seeds, fruits and vegetables

Learn More: Sport Nutrition Textbook pgs. 3-5

FIBER

- Comprised of non-digestible carbohydrates in plants, resists enzymatic action in the intestine
- Provides numerous physiological benefits, low caloric yield (mechanical/bacterial breakdown), and high satiety
- Recommended intake of 20 to 35 g/day
- **Insoluble fiber** – increases bulk and softens stool, shortens transit time through the intestine
  - Found in bran, nuts and seeds, many vegetables, skins of fruit
- **Soluble fiber** – undergoes metabolic action to yield many health benefits, shown to lower blood cholesterol and normalize blood glucose, fermentation helps maintain healthy bacteria in colon
  - Found in legumes, oats, rye, barley, some fruits, and root vegetables

Learn More: Sport Nutrition Textbook pgs. 5-7

LIPIDS

- **Dietary lipids** - oils, fats, waxes, cholesterol
- **Endogenous lipids** – fatty acids, triacylglycerols (triglycerides), lipoproteins, and phospholipids

Functions

1. Serve as an important energy source - particularly during rest and prolonged exercise
   - Fatty acids and triglycerides are only forms used directly for fuel
2. Protection of vital organs (visceral) and padding for joints and other structures (subcutaneous)
3. Aid in fat-soluble vitamin absorption and storage
4. Form cell membranes and various hormones
5. Transport molecules
6. Serve in temperature regulation

Learn More: Sport Nutrition Textbook pgs. 9-10, 13

CLASSES OF LIPIDS

Simple lipids	• Fuel - triglycerides • Insulation, padding, and protection -neutral fat
Compound lipids	• Cell membranes - phospholipids • Serum cholesterol - lipoproteins (LDL, HDL)
Derived lipids	• Fuel - fatty acids • Hormone synthesis, regulatory functions – steroid compounds

Learn More: Sport Nutrition Textbook pgs. 9-13

FATTY ACIDS

- Important source of fuel, yielding significant energy
- Fatty acids are identified by their hydrocarbon chain length (number of carbons) and the number and location of double bonds

<u>Fatty Acid Types</u>

1. **Saturated fatty acids** – have no double hydrogen bonds in hydrocarbon chain
   - Primarily found in animal food sources
   - Considered potential risk for cardiovascular disease (increase LDL-C)
2. **Unsaturated fatty acids** – have one or more double hydrogen bonds in hydrocarbon chain.
   - Not a risk factor for CVD
3. **Monounsaturated fatty acids** – have one double hydrogen bond in hydrocarbon chain
   - Found in many plant oils – canola, olive, safflower, sunflower
4. **Polyunsaturated fatty acids** – have two or more double hydrogen bonds in hydrocarbon chain
   - Includes the essential fatty acids that regulate various bodily functions (linoleic acid, α-linolenic acid), omega-3 and omega-6 fatty acids
   - Found in fatty fish, seed oils
5. **Trans fatty acids** – unsaturated fatty acids that have a modified chemical configuration (hydrogenation)
   - Considered useful for baking (high melting point) and dramatically extend shelf life of foods
   - Known to significantly increase cardiovascular disease risk by elevating serum LDL and lowering serum HDL

Learn More: Sport Nutrition Textbook pgs. 9-12

CHOLESTEROL

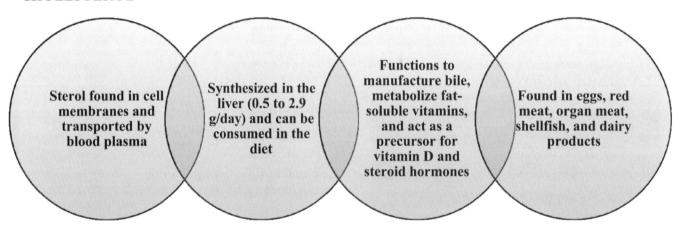

Sterol found in cell membranes and transported by blood plasma

Synthesized in the liver (0.5 to 2.9 g/day) and can be consumed in the diet

Functions to manufacture bile, metabolize fat-soluble vitamins, and act as a precursor for vitamin D and steroid hormones

Found in eggs, red meat, organ meat, shellfish, and dairy products

Learn More: Sport Nutrition Textbook pgs. 9 & 14

PROTEIN

- Provides structure to organs, connective tissue, muscle, skin, hair
- Comprised of amino acids (AA) bound by peptide bonds (polypeptides)
- **11 Nonessential amino acids** – can be internally synthesized
- **9 Essential amino acids** (EAA) – cannot be internally synthesized, must be derived from diet
- **Complete proteins** contain all of the EAAs - meat, poultry, fish, dairy, and soybean
- EAAs can be synthesized by combining certain **incomplete protein** sources such as rice and beans
- Basic nutrition recommends intake of 0.8 to 1.2g/kg for sedentary population, 10%-15% of total kcal consumed per day

Learn More: Sport Nutrition Textbook pgs. 15-18

WATER

- Adult body is about 60% water by weight, approximate content varies by tissue: blood – 90%, muscle – 75%, bone – 25%, adipose – 5%
- Typical adult needs 2.0 to 2.8 L/day (66 to 94 oz/day) based on activity levels and size

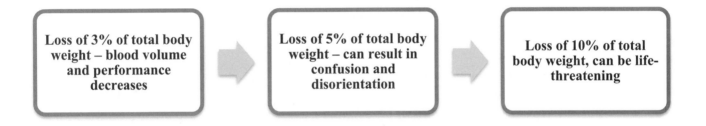

Loss of 3% of total body weight – blood volume and performance decreases → Loss of 5% of total body weight – can result in confusion and disorientation → Loss of 10% of total body weight, can be life-threatening

Functions

1. Transports nutrients and waste products
2. Regulates body temperature
3. Participates in biochemical reactions
4. Provides lubrication
5. Cleanses or protects joints and organs
6. Acts as a solvent to allow proper electrolyte dynamics

Learn More: Sport Nutrition Textbook pgs. 18-19

VITAMINS AND MINERALS

- Vitamins (organic), minerals, and trace elements (inorganic) aid in the metabolism of food products and numerous chemical reactions to maintain homeostasis
- 13 known essential vitamins – 9 water-soluble, 4 fat-soluble
- All must be obtained from the diet except for:
    o Vitamin D (synthesized from sunlight)
    o Vitamin K (synthesized by bacteria in intestines)
- **Macrominerals** require a daily intake >100 mg, **microminerals** require a daily intake <100 mg

    Learn More: Sport Nutrition Textbook pgs. 19-20

PHYTONUTRIENTS

- Organic components of plants thought to promote health benefits
- Not considered essential nutrients - no known nutritional deficiencies occur without intake
- Two classes that have received the most attention in research:
    o Carotenoids – found in red, orange and yellow pigmented fruits and vegetables
    o Polyphenols – found in various berries, fruits, wine, tea

Possible Mechanisms of Health Promotion

1. Antioxidant activity
2. Enhance the immune system
3. Alter hormonal balance
4. Conversion into vitamin A (beta-carotene)
5. Cause cancer cells to die
6. Repair DNA damage from toxic exposure

    Learn More: Sport Nutrition Textbook pgs. 20-22

Fat-Soluble and Water-Soluble Vitamins
Vitamin B_1 (thiamine)
Vitamin B_2 (riboflavin)
Vitamin B_3 (niacin)
Vitamin B_6 (pyridoxine)
Vitamin B_{12}
Biotin
Pantothenic acid
Folic acid
Vitamin C (ascorbic acid)
Vitamin A
Vitamin D
Vitamin E (alpha-tocopherol)
Vitamin K

SECTION 3   • <u>**REVIEW YOUR KNOWLEDGE**</u>

<u>Match the Following Terms</u>

1. _____ Starch   a. Provides 7 kcal per gram when consumed

2. _____ Bran   b. Is an essential fatty acid

3. _____ Micronutrients   c. Provides low caloric yield with high satiety

4. _____ Protein   d. Solvent to allow proper electrolyte dynamics

5. _____ Linoleic acid   e. Storage form of carbohydrate in plants

6. _____ Glycogen   f. Example of an insoluble fiber food source

7. _____ Phytonutrients   g. Storage form of carbohydrate in humans

8. _____ Fiber   h. Present in the diet in small quantities (<1g/day)

9. _____ Water   i. Can regulate metabolism in the form of enzymes

10. _____ Alcohol   j. Can serve as antioxidants

<u>Knowledge and Competency Exercises</u>

11. List the four categories of macronutrients.

a) _____   b) _____

c) _____   d)_____

12. List three primary functions of nutrients in the human body.

a) _____

b) _____

c) _____

13. _____ are known to promote cardiovascular disease by elevating LDL cholesterol and reducing HDL cholesterol.

14. Cholesterol can be consumed in the diet but is also synthesized in the _____ at a rate of 0.5 to 2.9 g/day.

15. True or False? *(circle one)* Proteins are comprised of numerous amino acids bound by peptide bonds.

16. Athletes are generally recommended to consume approximately _____ of their total energy intake in the form of healthy carbohydrates.

17. Identify two fat-soluble vitamins that are synthesized in the body.

a) _____   b) _____

18. List two common beverages that contain the class of phytonutrients known as polyphenols.

a) _____   b) _____

SECTION 4 • **ASSESS YOUR KNOWLEDGE**

1. Which of the following types of nutrients primarily serve to promote growth and development?

   a. Carbohydrates
   b. Fats
   c. Trace elements
   d. Proteins

2. Which of the following nutrients include the essential fatty acids?

   a. Saturated fatty acids
   b. Unsaturated fatty acids
   c. Polyunsaturated fatty acids
   d. Cholesterol

3. Which of the following nutrients is predominantly used during high-intensity training?

   a. Fats
   b. Carbohydrates
   c. Vitamins
   d. Proteins

4. Starch is an example of which of the following classes of carbohydrate?

   a. Monosaccharides
   b. Disaccharides
   c. Polysaccharides
   d. Fiber

5. Which of the following nutrients shorten transit time of waste products and potential toxins in the intestinal tract?

   a. Trans fatty acids
   b. Insoluble fiber
   c. Polypeptides
   d. Oligosaccharides

6. Which of the following forms of lipids can act as a precursor to vitamin D and the hormone testosterone?

  a. Medium-chain fatty acids
  b. Monounsaturated fat
  c. Cholesterol
  d. Saturated fat

7. Which of the following protein sources do not contain all of the essential amino acids?

  a. Wheat
  b. Beef
  c. Fish
  d. Egg

8. The recommended daily intake of protein for a sedentary individual is:

  a. 0.8 to 1.2g/kg of total body weight
  b. 30% of total caloric intake
  c. 1.5 to 2g/kg of total body weight
  d. 75g-100g

9. Which of the following is the only form of carbohydrate that can be directly oxidized in muscle tissue to fuel exercise?

  a. Sucrose
  b. Glucose
  c. Fructose
  d. Maltodextrin

10. Which of the following is not a mechanism by which phytonutrients aid in maintaining health?

  a. Strengthening of the immune system
  b. Altering of estrogen metabolism
  c. Conversion into vitamin K (carotenoids)
  d. Repairing of DNA damage as a result of toxic exposure such as smoking

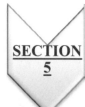

SECTION 5   • <u>**CHECK YOUR WORK**</u>

SPORT NUTRITION CHAPTER 1 ANSWERS

<u>MATCH THE FOLLOWING TERMS</u>

1. E	5. B	9. D
2. F	6. G	10. A
3. H	7. J	
4. I	8. C	

<u>KNOWLEDGE AND COMPETENCY EXERCISES</u>

11. Carbohydrate, Fat, Protein, Water

12. Promotion of growth and development, provision of energy, regulation of metabolism

13. Trans fatty acids

14. Liver

15. True

16. 60%

17. Vitamin D, Vitamin K

18. Tea, Wine

<u>ASSESS YOUR KNOWLEDGE</u>

1. D	5. B	9. B
2. C	6. C	10. C
3. B	7. A	
4. C	8. A	

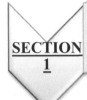

SECTION 1 • LEARNING GOALS

Upon completing this section, along with its corresponding chapter, you should understand the following:

1. The definitions and intended uses of recommended nutrient intake values such as the DRI, EAR, RDA, AI, UL, DV, and DRV

2. The development of the initial RDA values and recommendations into the current standards

3. Practical guidelines for healthy eating based on data from major organizations and programs such as the USDA

4. The specific recommendations found in the MyPyramid nutritional education guide

5. The recommendations for daily intake of carbohydrate, fat, and protein

6. How to properly assess the nutritional quality of food by examining the nutrition facts label

7. The definitions of common nutrient content claims or descriptions

8. The criteria that must be met for a food product to make a specific health claim on the label

9. The methods of food processing and the effects on the original product

10. Examples and uses of food additives and artificial ingredients

11. The common methods for estimating nutrient intake

SECTION 2 • **QUICKFACTS**

ESSENTIAL AND NON-ESSENTIAL NUTRIENTS

- Humans require 46 **essential nutrients**
- **Non-essential nutrients** can be synthesized in the body from their precursors; they are not directly required in the diet

> **A nutrient is considered essential if:**
>
> • It is required in the diet for growth, health, and overall survival
> • Absence or inadequate intake results in signs of a deficiency disease
> • Growth failure and signs of deficiency are prevented only by the nutrient or a specific precursor of the nutrient
> • Below the critical level of necessary intake for the given nutrient, growth response and severity of signs of deficiency are proportional to the amount consumed
> • It is not synthesized in the body and is required for a critical function throughout life

Learn More: Sport Nutrition Textbook pgs 26-27

DEFINING RECOMMENDED NUTRIENT INTAKE VALUES

- **Dietary Reference Intake (DRI)** – New standards for nutrient recommendations that can be used to plan and assess diets for healthy people
- **Estimated Average Requirements (EAR)** – Nutrient intake value that is estimated to meet the requirement of 50% of the healthy individuals in a group, used to assess nutritional adequacy of intakes of population groups and to calculate RDAs
- **Recommended Dietary Allowance (RDA)** – A daily dietary intake level that is sufficient to meet the nutrient requirement of 97-98% of all healthy people in a group; if an EAR cannot be set, no RDA can be proposed
- **Adequate Intake (AI)** – Value used when no RDA can be determined, recommended daily intake level based on research-based approximation of intake for a group of healthy people
- **Tolerable Upper Intake Level (UL)** – Highest level of daily nutrient intake that is likely to pose no risks or adverse health effects to almost all individuals in the general population, as intake increases above the UL the risk of adverse effects increases

Learn More: Sport Nutrition Textbook pg 28

DEVELOPMENT OF CURRENT RDA VALUES

- First set of RDA values created in 1941 by the **Food and Nutrition Board** to prevent diseases caused by nutrient deficiencies
  - ➢ Included reference values for only 10 nutrients
  - ➢ Developed to evaluate and plan nutritional adequacy of large groups such as the armed forces and children in school lunch programs
  - ➢ Designed to prevent deficiency in vast majority of a population – but not to meet the specific needs of individuals
- Revised several times until current DRI guidelines established between 1997-2004
  - ➢ Now includes 46 nutrients
  - ➢ Incorporates values such as EAR, AI, and UL to meet individual and group needs
  - ➢ Also aimed at reducing the risk of diet-related chronic conditions (e.g., heart disease, diabetes, hypertension, osteoporosis) and meeting specific needs among genders and age groups (e.g., children, pregnant women)

Learn More: Sport Nutrition Textbook pgs 27-28

CLOSER LOOK AT CURRENT INTAKE VALUES

- RDA
  - ➢ Cannot be set without an established EAR, is a safe 'excess' level above the set EAR
  - ➢ Meals in institutions are considered adequate if nutrient levels fall between RDA and EAR
  - ➢ Currently available for energy intake, protein, 11 vitamins, and 7 minerals

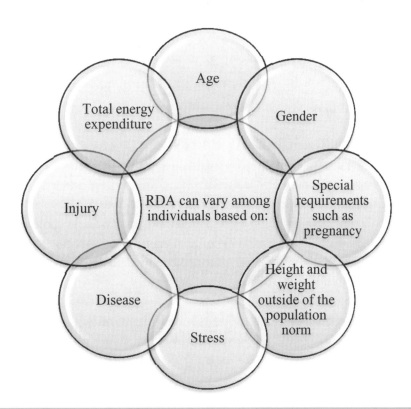

- AI
  - ➢ Represents a mean intake that appears to sustain a desired indicator of health (e.g. calcium retention in bone)
  - ➢ Has been set for two B vitamins, choline, vitamin D, and a number of minerals
- UL
  - ➢ Not intended to represent recommended intake but rather indicate a potentially toxic level
  - ➢ Developed after the increased practice of fortifying foods and popularity of dietary supplements which present greater risk of adverse effects compared to natural sources

Learn More: Sport Nutrition Textbook pgs 28-30

MYPYRAMID

- Developed by the **United States Department of Agriculture (USDA)** from an antiquated food guide pyramid to provide practical dietary guidance
- Distinguishes six food groups to ensure a balanced nutrient intake:

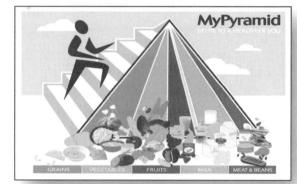

  - ➢ Bread, cereal, rice, and pasta
  - ➢ Vegetables
  - ➢ Milk, yogurt, and cheese
  - ➢ Fruits
  - ➢ Meat, poultry, fish, eggs, dry beans, and nuts
  - ➢ Fats, oils, and sweets
- Adult recommendations: **45-65% of energy from carbohydrates, 20-35% of energy from fat, 10-35% from protein**
- Has a supporting website that aids in developing individualized food plans and assessing nutrient intake - www.mypyramidtracker.gov/

Learn More: Sport Nutrition Textbook pg 32-33

PRACTICAL GUIDELINES FOR HEALTHY EATING

1. Balance food intake with physical activity to maintain a healthy weight
2. Eat a variety of nutrient-rich foods
3. Eat a diet rich in vegetables, fruits, and whole-grain and high-fiber foods
4. Choose a diet moderate in total fat but low in saturated fat, trans fat, and cholesterol
   - ➢ Keep saturated fatty acids below 10% of total energy intake
   - ➢ Keep trans fat intake to less than 1% of total energy intake
   - ➢ Limit cholesterol intake to 300 mg or less per day
   - ➢ Choose low-fat or fat-free dairy products
5. Cut back on beverages and foods high in calories and low in nutrition
   - ➢ Cut back on soft drinks and foods with added sugar
   - ➢ Attempt to cut processed or added sugars to 10% or less of total energy intake
6. Keep salt and sodium intake conservative
7. Drink alcohol in moderation

> ➤ Non-nutrient but provides 7 kcal/g
> ➤ Research suggests that moderate intake poses no negative health effects, one drink a day for women, up to two drinks a day for men

8. Practice food hygiene and safety
9. Avoid excessive intake of food additives and nutrition supplements

Learn More: Sport Nutrition Textbook pgs 34-35

FOOD LABEL VALUES

- Designed to help consumers make choices by providing detailed information concerning the nutrient content of the food product and how it fits into an overall diet
- **Nutrition Labeling and Education Act of 1990** standardized US food labels
- **Daily Values (DV)** - developed by **the Food and Drug Administration (FDA)** by condensing **U.S. RDA** values (also known as **Reference Daily Intake (RDI)** values) into acceptable recommendations for all groups to simplify label data
- **Daily Reference Value (DRV)** – standard for dietary components that have no RDA
  - ➤ Includes total fat, saturated fat, cholesterol, total carbohydrate, fiber, sodium, potassium, and protein
- **"% Daily Value"** - percentage of the RDA or DRV (as applicable) available in a single serving

Learn More: Sport Nutrition Textbook pg 30 & 35

Macaroni & cheese

Nutrition Facts

Serving Size 1 cup (228g)
Serving Per Container 2

Amount Per Serving

Calories 250	Calories from Fat 110

% Daily Value*

Total Fat 12g	18%
Saturated Fat 3g	15%
Cholesterol 30mg	10%
Sodium 470mg	20%
Total Carbohydrate 31g	10%
Dietary Fiber 0g	0%
Sugars 5g	
Protein 5g	

Vitamin A	4%
Vitamin C	2%
Calcium	20%
Iron	4%

*Percent Daily Values are based on a 2,000 calorie diet. Your Daily Values may be higher or lower depending on your calorie needs:

	Calories	2,000	2,500
Total Fat	Less than	65g	80g
Sat Fat	Less than	20g	25g
Cholesterol	Less than	300mg	300mg
Sodium	Less than	2,400mg	2,400mg
Total Carbohydrate		300g	375g
Dietary Fiber		25g	30g

Start here —

Limit these nutrients

5% or less is low

20% or more is high

Get enough of these nutrients

Footnote

© 2010 Human Kinetics

UNDERSTANDING FOOD LABELS

- Nutrition Facts Label will include:
  - ➤ Serving size and serving per package
  - ➤ Calories per serving and calories from fat
  - ➤ Quantity of key nutrients (in grams or milligrams) and reflective % Daily Value based on a 2,000 calorie diet
    - ▪ Nutrients that should be limited – total fat, saturated fat, cholesterol, sodium
    - ▪ Total carbohydrates – divided into fiber and sugar content
    - ▪ Protein
    - ▪ Key vitamins and minerals
  - ➤ Footnote information describing optimal nutrient intake for 2,000 and 2,500 calorie diets as well as the calories provided per gram for fat, carbohydrate, and protein

Learn More: Sport Nutrition Textbook pgs 35-36

FOOD PRODUCT CONTENT CLAIMS

- Many labels contain food descriptors with definitions that are regulated by the FDA, but commonly misunderstood by consumers
  - ➢ Free – calorie free, fat free, sugar free
  - ➢ Low – low calorie, low fat
  - ➢ Reduced – reduced calories, reduced fat, reduced sugar
  - ➢ Light, lean, fresh, pure, 100%, etc.
- See Table 2.3 on page 37 for detailed definitions of common descriptors or content claims

Learn More: Sport Nutrition Textbook pgs 36-37

FOOD PRODUCT HEALTH CLAIMS

- Many labels contain statements about the beneficial effects of the food product on the body (e.g. "Helps maintain a healthy heart" or "Aids in digestion")
- Claims must:
  - ➢ Be based on scientific evidence such as epidemiological studies
  - ➢ Include an explanation about why the food is beneficial
  - ➢ Include a % DV for the beneficial ingredient(s) in the product
    - ▪ Must be a naturally good source (≥10%)
    - ▪ Must not contain >20% of the DV for fat, saturated fat, cholesterol, or sodium
- Must also include a disclaimer that the food cannot treat, prevent, or cure any disease or medical condition as these claims only apply to regulated medicines
- See Table 2.4 on page 38 for descriptions of legal health claims regulated by the FDA

Learn More: Sport Nutrition Textbook pgs 37-38

PROCESSED FOODS

- Refers to food treated to extend storage life or improve taste, nutritional value, color, or texture
- Can significantly reduce nutritional quality and biochemistry of the food
  - ➢ Example: bleaching of flour destroys 22 known essential nutrients in the original product

Learn More: Sport Nutrition Textbook pgs 37-38

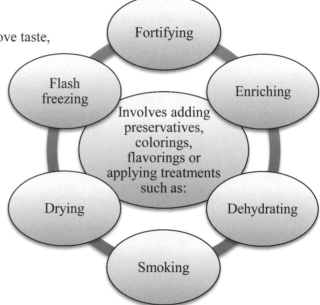

FOOD ADDITIVES AND ARTIFICIAL INGREDIENTS

- **Food additives** - lengthen shelf life, enhance color, texture or taste, facilitate food preparation, or otherwise make the product more marketable
  - ➤ Sugar and salt are common, economical preservatives
  - ➤ Food color additives commonly used to make food more appealing or appear fresh
- **Artificial ingredients** – synthetically derived, may contain few or no nutrients, may have the same quantity of energy as their natural counterparts
  - ➤ Non-dairy creamers, synthetic fruit juices
- **Artificial sweeteners** commonly contain no calories and generally provide a degree of sweetness that surpasses natural sugar
  - ➤ Saccharin, aspartame, sorbitol, sucralose, stevia extract

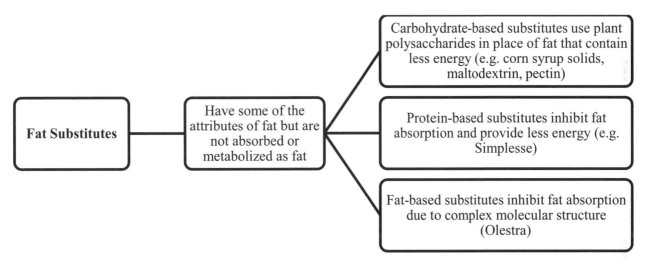

Learn More: Sport Nutrition Textbook pgs 38-40

ANALYZING DIETARY INTAKE

- There are many methods for assessing food intake and diet composition that differ in their accuracy and practicality
- Prospective methods:
  - ➤ 3-day dietary survey – Record food consumed for 3 days
  - ➤ 3-day weighed food record – Weigh and record food consumed for 3 days
  - ➤ 7-day dietary survey – Record food consumed for 7 days
  - ➤ 7-day weighed food record – Weigh and record food consumed for 7 days
  - ➤ Duplicate food collections – Save a duplicate of food for chemical analysis
- Retrospective methods:
  - ➤ 24-hour recall – questionnaire to assess intake in previous 24 hrs; most common method
  - ➤ Food frequency – questionnaire focusing on the frequency of intake of certain foods
  - ➤ Diet history – combines 24-hour recall and food frequency methods

Learn More: Sport Nutrition Textbook pgs 40-44

SECTION 3 • REVIEW YOUR KNOWLEDGE

Match the Following Terms

1. _____ DV

2. _____ Potassium

3. _____ 7-day dietary survey

4. _____ Aspartame

5. _____ AI

6. _____ Trans fat

7. _____ UL

8. _____ Olestra

9. _____ EAR

10. _____ 24-hour recall

a. A sucrose polymer-based fat substitute

b. Used when a RDA value cannot be determined

c. Should be less than 1% of total energy intake

d. Meets the nutrient need for 50% of people in a group

e. Has a DRV of 3,500 mg

f. A prospective method for estimating nutrient intake

g. Synthetic additive with 180x the sweetness of sucrose

h. Used on food labels to represent a simple RDA value

i. A retrospective method for estimating nutrient intake

j. Highest level of safe daily intake for a given nutrient

Knowledge and Competency Exercises

11. List two criteria for a nutrient to be considered essential.

a) _____

b) _____

12. True or False? *(circle one)* The RDA is a safe excess of nutrients above the EAR that prevents nutritional deficiencies in 97-98% of all healthy people in a given group.

13. True or False? *(circle one)* The current DRI guidelines include 58 essential nutrients.

14. According to the established daily reference values, saturated fat consumption should equal no more than _____ of total energy intake.

15. The UL for daily nutrient intake was developed after the increased practice of _____ foods and the popularity of _____.

16. According to the *2005 Dietary Guidelines for Americans*, _____ of energy intake should come from carbohydrate and _____ of energy intake should come from protein.

17. List five practical guidelines for healthy eating.

a) _____

b) _____

c) _____

d) _____

e) _____

18. True or False? *(circle one)* Stevia is an artificial sweetener derived from an herbal plant extract.

19. Fill in the following table covering common nutrient content claims found on food product labels.

Claim on Label	Calories	Total Fat	Sugars
'Free'	Less than 5 calories per serving		
'Low'			Not defined; no basis for recommended intake
'Reduced'		At least 25% less fat per serving than reference	

20. The _____ technique of estimating nutrient intake involves direct chemical analysis of all food products consumed during a given period, making it an especially accurate method.

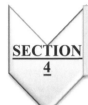

• PRACTICAL APPLICATIONS

CASE STUDY 1 – READING A FOOD LABEL

The following food labels belong to a can of spaghetti and meatballs in tomato sauce (left) and a carton of organic soy milk (right). For lunch, Sally prepared and consumed the entire can of spaghetti and meatballs and two cups of the organic soy milk. Review the labels and answer the questions that follow about the nutritional satisfaction of the meal.

Nutrition Facts		Nutrition Facts	
Serving Size 1 cup		Serving Size 1 cup	
Servings Per Container 2		Servings Per Container 4	
Amount Per Serving		**Amount Per Serving**	
Calories 270	Calories from Fat 90	Calories 100	Calories from Fat 36
	% Daily Value*		% Daily Value*
Total Fat 10g	15%	Total Fat 4g	6%
Saturated Fat 4.5g	23%	Saturated Fat 0.5g	3%
Cholesterol 20mg	7%	Cholesterol 0mg	0%
Sodium 900mg	38%	Sodium 110mg	5%
Total Carbohydrates 32g	11%	Total Carbohydrates 8g	3%
Fiber 2g	8%	Dietary Fiber 1g	4%
Sugars 8g		Sugars 6g	
Protein 11g		Protein 8g	
Vitamin A 6%	Vitamin C 0%	Vitamin A 5%	Vitamin C 0%
Calcium 2%	Iron 10%	Calcium 25%	Iron 6%

*Percent Values are based on a 2,000 calorie diet. Your Daily values may be higher or lower depending on your calorie needs:			*Percent Values are based on a 2,000 calorie diet. Your Daily values may be higher or lower depending on your calorie needs:		
	Calories	2,000		Calories	2,000
Total fat	Less than	65g	Total fat	Less than	65g
Sat fat	Less than	20g	Sat fat	Less than	20g
Cholesterol	Less than	300mg	Cholesterol	Less than	300mg
Sodium	Less than	2,400mg	Sodium	Less than	2,400mg
Total Carbohydrates		300g	Total Carbohydrates		300g
Fiber		25g	Fiber		25g
Calories per gram:			Calories per gram:		
Fat 9 Carbohydrate 4 Protein 4			Fat 9 Carbohydrate 4 Protein 4		

1. What is a single serving size for each of the food products consumed?
    Spaghetti and meatballs _____
    Organic Soy Milk _____
2. What was the total number of servings reportedly consumed?
    Spaghetti and meatballs _____
    Organic Soy Milk _____

3. What was the total number of calories consumed? _____

4. How many of the calories consumed came from fat? _____

5. What percentage of the total calories came from fat? _____ (fat kcal ÷ total kcal)

6. What percentage of the fat calories came from saturated fat? _____ (sat.fat kcal ÷ total fat kcal)

7. How many of the calories consumed came from carbohydrates? _____

8. What percentage of the total calories came from carbohydrates? _____ (CHO kcal ÷ total kcal)

9. How many grams of fiber were consumed? _____

10. What percentage of the total calories came from sugar? _____ (Sugar kcal ÷ total kcal)

11. How many of the calories consumed came from protein? _____

12. What percentage of the total calories came from protein? _____ (Protein kcal ÷ total kcal)

CASE STUDY 2 – UNDERSTANDING NUTRIENT NEEDS

Johnny currently plays collegiate football, which demands his participation in intense strength training approximately four days per week as well as conditioning two days per week during the offseason. The registered dietician in the athletic department recommended that he maintain adequate energy and consume 20% of calories from lean protein for recovery from the training. Due to the intensity and volume of his offseason training, and his calculated metabolic rate, the dietician suggests he take in approximately 3,300 kcal per day for optimal recovery and growth. Answer the following questions based on Johnny's specific nutrient needs.

1. How many daily kcal should Johnny consume in the form of protein? _____

2. How many daily grams of protein would this equate to? _____

• ASSESS YOUR KNOWLEDGE

SECTION 5

1. Which of the following is not considered an essential nutrient?

   a. Calcium
   b. Tryptophan
   c. Choline
   d. Vitamin D

2. Which of the following includes the new standards for nutrient recommendations that can be used to plan and assess diets for healthy people?

   a. UL
   b. DRI
   c. EAR
   d. AI

3. The current nutrient intake recommendations differ from the initial set developed in 1941 in which of the following ways?

   a. They are aimed at being able to develop and evaluate nutritional adequacy of large groups such as the armed forces
   b. They now include 27 essential nutrients
   c. They now meet the nutritional needs of 100% of healthy adults
   d. They are aimed at reducing the risk of diet-related chronic conditions such as diabetes, hypertension, heart disease, and osteoporosis

4. What percentile range of the total diet among healthy adults should come from fat, based on the updated *2005 Dietary Guidelines for Americans*?

   a. 10-20%
   b. 15-25%
   c. 20-35%
   d. 30-40%

5. Which of the following food groups from the MyPyramid nutritional guidance tool provided by the U.S. government serves as a good source of iron?

   a. Fruit
   b. Meat, poultry, fish, eggs, dry beans, nuts
   c. Dairy products: milk, yogurt, cheese
   d. Fats, oils, sweets

6. It is recommended that the daily intake of dietary cholesterol not surpass which of the following quantities?

 a. 100mg
 b. 150mg
 c. 300mg
 d. 415mg

7. When examining nutrition facts on the label of a food product, which of the following nutrients is listed toward the top of the label as it is a nutrient that is recommended to be limited in the diet?

 a. Dietary fiber
 b. Sodium
 c. Vitamin A
 d. Protein

8. Which of the following health claims may be presented on a food product that provides ≥10% of the Daily Value for folic acid?

 a. The product may claim to reduce the risk for dental caries
 b. The product may claim to reduce the risk for certain types of cancer
 c. The product may claim to reduce the risk for birth defects
 d. The product may claim to reduce the risk for heart disease

9. Which of the following artificial sweeteners provides the same caloric yield per gram as sucrose but, considering it is only used in minute amounts, adds virtually no energy to a given food source?

 a. Saccharin
 b. Aspartame
 c. Sorbitol
 d. Xylitol

10. Which of the following techniques for estimating nutrient intake is essentially a combination of the processes implemented in the 24-hour recall and food frequency methods?

 a. Diet history method
 b. Duplicate food collections method
 c. 3-day dietary survey
 d. 7-day weighed food record

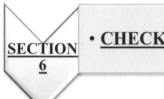

SPORT NUTRITION CHAPTER 2 ANSWERS

<u>**MATCH THE FOLLOWING TERMS**</u>

1. H	5. B	9. D
2. E	6. C	10. I
3. F	7. J	
4. G	8. A	

<u>**KNOWLEDGE AND COMPETENCY EXERCISES**</u>

11. Possible choices: **a)** The substance is required in the diet for growth, health, and overall survival, **b)** Absence or inadequate intake of the substance results in signs of a deficiency disease and ultimately death, **c)** Growth failure and signs of deficiency are prevented only by the nutrient or a specific precursor of it, **d)** Below the critical level of necessary intake for the given nutrient, growth response and severity of signs of deficiency are proportional to the amount consumed, **e)** The substance is not synthesized in the body and is required for a critical function throughout life

12. True

13. False

14. 10%

15. Fortifying, dietary supplements

16. 45-65%, 10-35%

17. Possible choices: **a)** Balance food intake with physical activity to maintain a healthy weight, **b)** Eat a variety of nutrient-rich foods, **c)** Eat a diet rich in vegetables, fruits, and whole-grain and high-fiber foods, **d)** Choose a diet moderate in total fat but low in saturated fat, trans fat, and cholesterol, **e)** Cut back on beverages and foods high in calories and low in nutrition, **f)** Keep salt and sodium intake conservative, **g)** Drink alcohol in moderation, **h)** Practice food hygiene and safety, **i)** Avoid excessive intake of food additives and nutrition supplements

18. True

19.

Claim on Label	Calories	Total Fat	Sugars
'Free'	Less than 5 calories per serving	*Less than 0.5 grams per reference amount*	*Less than 0.5 grams per reference amount*
'Low'	*40 calories or less per reference amount*	*3 grams or less per reference amount*	Not defined; no basis for recommended intake
'Reduced'	*25% fewer calories per serving than reference*	25% less fat per serving than reference	*25% less sugar per serving than reference*

20. Duplicate food collections

CASE STUDY 1

1. Spaghetti and meatballs – 1 cup, organic soy milk – 1 cup

2. Spaghetti and meatballs - 2 organic soy milk - 2

3. 740 kcal

4. 252 kcal

5. 34%

6. 35.7%

7. 320 kcal

8. 43.2%

9. 6g

10. 15.1%

11. 152 kcal

12. 20.5%

CASE STUDY 2

1. 660 kcal

2. 165g

ASSESS YOUR KNOWLEDGE

1. C

2. B

3. D

4. C

5. B

6. C

7. B

8. C

9. B

10. A

SECTION 1   • <u>LEARNING GOALS</u>

Upon completing this section, along with its corresponding chapter, you should understand the following:

1. **How skeletal muscle fibers produce force**

2. **The cascade of events involved in skeletal muscle contraction and relaxation**

3. **The characteristics of different muscle fiber types and variability within different muscle tissue**

4. **The anaerobic and aerobic systems of metabolism that function to produce energy (ATP)**

5. **How energy is stored and used for work in the body**

6. **The hormones involved in regulating energy metabolism during exercise and stress**

7. **Factors that can affect the metabolic responses to exercise**

8. **The causes of fatigue for varying exercise intensities and durations**

9. **The metabolic adaptations that occur with aerobic and anaerobic exercise**

• **QUICKFACTS**

WHY UNDERSTAND BASIC BIOCHEMISTRY?

- Helps to explain a number of practical applications of sport nutrition and exercise such as:
  - o Appropriate rest periods and work-to-rest ratios
  - o Energy needs for varying types of training
  - o Causes of short-term or prolonged fatigue
- Biochemistry refers to the study of:
  - o Cellular and enzymatic reactions
  - o Energy transfer
  - o Hormonal effects of exercise
  - o Transport processes at sub-cellular and molecular levels
- Refer to Appendix A for extra study on principles of biochemistry and cell biology

Learn More: Sport Nutrition Textbook pgs 48, 395-414

MUSCLE STRUCTURE UNDER THE MICROSCOPE

- Muscle tissue is comprised of long, cylindrical cells called fibers which contain organelles and structures that allow for contraction and relaxation
- Structures inside fibers:
  - o **Sarcoplasm** – cell cytoplasm that stores energy as fat, glycogen, **phosphocreatine (PCr)** and **adenosine triphosphate (ATP)**
  - o **Mitochondria** – energy producing organelles
  - o **Myoglobin** – intracellular oxygen carrier
  - o Myofibrils – filaments that give muscle its striated appearance under microscope
    - ▪ **Actin** – thin myofilament
    - ▪ **Myosin** – thick myofilament

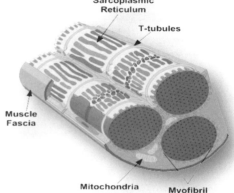

- **Sarcoplasmic reticulum (SR) -** surrounds myofibrils and store calcium ions for contraction
- **Sarcomere** – repeating contractile unit of a muscle fiber that shortens during contraction

Learn More: Sport Nutrition Textbook pg 48-49

SKELETAL MUSCLE CONTRACTION

1. Nerve stimulus sends electrical excitation in the form of an **action potential** to cell membrane
2. Action potential travels down **T-tubules** to stimulate release of calcium from the SR
3. Calcium ions released from the SR bind to the regulatory protein **troponin,** which in turn causes the regulatory filament **tropomyosin** to move away from potential **binding sites** on actin
4. After binding site is uncovered, myosin can connect to actin to form **cross-bridges**
5. **Power strokes** of myosin heads at cross-bridges pull actin toward the center of sarcomeres, causing the muscle to shorten and a consequent contraction
   a. Breakdown of ATP on myosin heads by enzyme **ATPase** causes an energy release to fuel the power strokes (much like an oar stroke in a boat)
   b. **Adenosine diphosphate (ADP)** and an **inorganic phosphate (Pi)** are released from ATP metabolism
6. As a new ATP molecule binds to the myosin head, the head detaches and the cycle repeats itself
   a. Cross-bridges repeatedly attach and detach in a rapid fashion allowing for fluid, continuous shortening of the muscle

Learn More: Sport Nutrition Textbook pgs 48-49

SKELETAL MUSCLE RELAXATION

Contraction is inhibited by insufficient ATP or calcium, or an environment that is not conducive to energy metabolism (e.g. disruption of ATPase due to acidic environment)

⇩

Calcium pump in SR draws calcium back into storage to produce muscle fiber relaxation

⇩

Tropomyosin returns to position that blocks binding sites on actin

Learn More: Sport Nutrition Textbook pg 49

MUSCLE FIBER TYPES

- **Type I fibers** – slow twitch fibers
  - Small diameter, slow-acting myosin ATPase activity and therefore slow contraction rate; high myoglobin, mitochondria, and capillary density allow for a rich supply of oxygen, nutrients, and energy; high capacity for oxidative metabolism; fatigue resistant
  - Specialized for repeated submaximal contractions for long periods of time
- **Type IIa fibers** – fast twitch, fatigue-resistant fibers

- - o Metabolic properties of both type I and type IIx, have fast-acting myosin ATPase activity and contractile speed similar to type IIx with oxidative capacity similar to type I fibers giving them moderate resistance to fatigue
  - **Type IIx fibers** – fast twitch, fatigable fibers
    - o Largest diameter, fast-acting myosin ATPase activity and therefore fast contraction rate; low myoglobin, mitochondria, and capillary density resulting in rapid fatigue and lactic acid accumulation; have greater glycogen and PCr stores that allow for rapid, powerful contractions for brief periods of time
  - Recruitment is based on need:

| Type I | ⇒ | Type IIa | ⇒ | Type IIx |

- - Low-intensity efforts use mostly type I, moderate-intensity efforts use type I and type IIa, maximal-intensity efforts use all three types

Learn More: Sport Nutrition Textbook pg 49-51

MUSCLE FIBER COMPOSITION
- Muscles contain all three fiber types in varying proportions based on function
  - o Postural muscles have high proportion of type I; i.e., the soleus
  - o Musculature that must produce rapid movements have a greater proportion of type II such as in the hand or around the eye
  - o Muscles such as the quadriceps may have a greater proportion of either type depending on genetics and training stimuli
    - ▪ Successful marathon runners – 80% type I in vastus lateralis
    - ▪ Elite sprinters – 60% type II in vastus lateralis
- The metabolic properties of fibers can be slightly modified, but fiber type cannot be changed
- Ultimately the density of a fiber type is genetically determined – sports pick the athletes based on physical aptitude

Learn More: Sport Nutrition Textbook pg 51

ENERGY FOR MUSCLE FORCE PRODUCTION
- ATP - source of energy for all muscular work
  Resting concentration of ATP can only fuel seconds of maximal exercise (e.g., 1RM); must be continually synthesized
- Three mechanisms involved in resynthesis of ATP:
  - o **PCr hydrolysis** – initial anaerobic process
  - o **Glycolysis** – secondary anaerobic process
  - o **Tricarboxylic acid (TCA) cycle** (Krebs Cycle) – aerobic process

Learn More: Sport Nutrition Textbook pg 51

NEW ATP THROUGH PHOSPHOCREATINE METABOLISM

- Provides rapid, but relatively limited, energy release without the need for oxygen; occurs in sarcoplasm of muscle cells
- PCr is broken down into creatine and P_i by the enzyme **creatine kinase (CK)** releasing free energy and donating the P_i to circulating ADP to reform new ATP

PCr (CK) → Creatine + P_i + Energy   »»»»»»   Energy + P_i + ADP → New ATP

- Provides energy that is sufficient to fuel short duration, high-intensity exercise such as sprints, or intense efforts at the onset of exercise; not a major contributor to prolonged activity

Learn More: Sport Nutrition Textbook pgs 51-53

GLYCOLYSIS IN ANAEROBIC METABOLISM

- Energy provided without the use of oxygen from the breakdown of glucose in blood and/or glycogen in muscle
- Actions occur in what is called the **glycolytic pathway** – involves a complex set of enzymatic reactions which break down sugars to form ATP and energy metabolites
- Released **hydrogen ions (H+)** during glucose breakdown lower the pH level in muscle

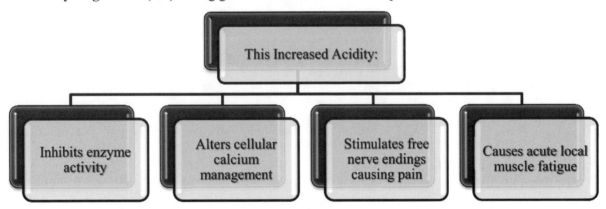

- Allows for the continuation of high-intensity, shorter duration work after PCr cannot sustain energy needs; for prolonged durations must work with aerobic metabolism

Learn More: Sport Nutrition Textbook pgs 53-56

AEROBIC METABOLISM

- Carbohydrates, fats, and proteins can be metabolized with the use of oxygen in the mitochondria to produce significant ATP for sustaining prolonged activity
- **Carbohydrates – Pyruvate** (byproduct of glucose metabolism) is used to form **acetyl-CoA** which in turn enters the TCA or Krebs cycle to produce ATP

- **Fats** – Lipolysis - Hormonal breakdown of fat stores provides **fatty acids (FA)** and glycerol
  - FA are metabolized through **β-oxidation** to form acetyl-CoA to produce ATP in the same manner as carbohydrates (TCA Cycle)
- **Proteins** – Amino acids are broken down by separating the amino group from a carbon skeleton (or keto-acid) to form acetyl-CoA to produce ATP in the same manner as carbohydrates or fats (TCA Cycle), or through other unique reactions
  - Becomes an increasingly important source during starvation or when glycogen stores are significantly depleted (no carb or low carb diet), causing the body to move from protein-sparing to glycogen-sparing mechanism

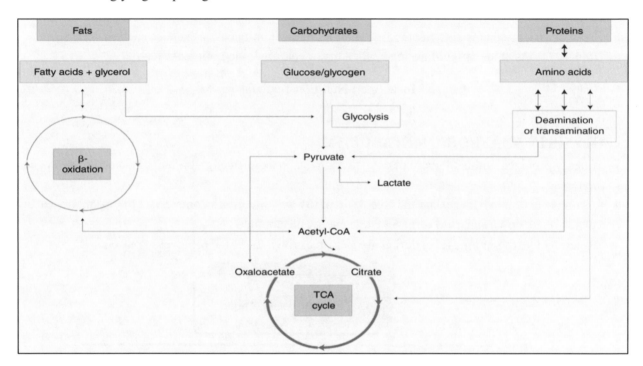

Learn More: Sport Nutrition Textbook pgs 56-62

ENERGY STORES FOR EXERCISE

- **Carbohydrates** are stored in the liver, skeletal muscle and blood
  - Skeletal muscle – as glycogen, approximately 13-18g/kg of body weight (300g available in the legs for events such as running or cycling)
  - Blood – as glucose
  - Liver – as glycogen, approximately 100g
  - Glycogen stores are normally depleted after 1-2 hours of intense exercise, causing significant performance decline
- **Fats** are stored in adipose tissue, and skeletal muscle
  - Adipose – Triglycerides undergo lipolysis to release FA into circulation for uptake
  - Skeletal muscle – contains approximately 12g/kg of body weight in the form of intramuscular triglycerides
  - Total fat stores could fuel an extremely prolonged period of exercise

- Fat stores provide more energy than carbohydrates per gram, but are used at a rate that can maintain an exercise intensity up to only about 60% VO_2max; for higher intensities carbohydrates must be used

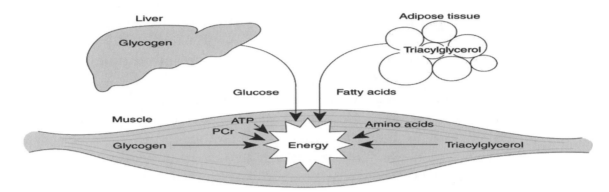

- **Protein** is not a primary energy nutrient, stores are minimal and therefore do not exceed 10% of daily energy usage under normal conditions

Learn More: Sport Nutrition Textbook pgs 62-63

REGULATION OF ENERGY METABOLISM

- Intramuscular energy is maintained by:
1. **Regulatory actions within muscle cells**
    a. Variances in ATP and its byproducts ADP, AMP, P_i ratios cause enzymatic reactions which function to rebalance ratio back to neutral state
    b. ATP, ADP and AMP concentrations also activate or inhibit the use of PCr, carbohydrates, or fats
    c. An increase in $Ca2^+$ levels due to muscular contraction increases energy uptake
2. **Sympathetic nervous system (SNS)**
    a. Stimulates the release of intramuscular energy sources via hormonal actions
3. **Hormones**
    a. **Insulin** – stimulates glucose and muscle amino acid uptake and storage, inhibits lipolysis and protein breakdown in response to a rise in blood glucose
    b. **Glucagon** – stimulates liver glycogen breakdown and **gluconeogenesis** (production of new glucose) in response to a fall in blood glucose
    c. **Epinephrine and Norepinephrine** – stimulates glycogen breakdown and lipolysis in response to stress and a fall in blood glucose
    d. **Cortisol** – stimulates protein breakdown for gluconeogenesis; stimulates lipolysis in response to stress
    e. **Growth hormone** – stimulates lipolysis in response to stress
    f. **Interleukin-6** – a muscle cytokine that stimulates liver glycogen breakdown, lipolysis, and cortisol secretion

Learn More: Sport Nutrition Textbook pgs 63-68

FACTORS THAT AFFECT THE METABOLIC RESPONSE TO EXERCISE

- Many factors can have an effect on the metabolic responses to exercise including:
    1. **Exercise intensity** – dictates predominant energy type used and rate of use
    2. **Exercise duration** – dictates predominant energy type used and storage depletion
    3. **Fitness level** – dictates capacity to use specific energy sources
    4. **Nutritional status** – determines pre-exercise storage; starvation promotes protein use
    5. **Diet** – availability of specific energy source affect use
    6. **Feeding during exercise** – carbohydrate intake can increase capacity
    7. **Mode of exercise** – isolated muscle exercise can cause acute glycogen depletion
    8. **Previous exercise** – glycogen depletion
    9. **Drugs or supplements** – creatine supplementation can enhance PCr system
    10. **Environmental temperature and altitude** – differing levels of stress

Learn More: Sport Nutrition Textbook pg 69

ENERGY METABOLISM AND FATIGUE

- **Fatigue** – inability to maintain a given or expected force or power output

<u>High Intensity Exercise</u>

- **During maximal, short-duration exercise** – fatigue caused by depletion of PCr and a rapid rate of glycolysis
- **During high-intensity exercise lasting 1 to 5 min** – fatigue caused by lactic acid accumulation
    o Lactic acid breaks down into lactate and H^+; increased muscle acidity from H^+ inhibits enzyme actions for energy production
    o Calcium transport from the SR is also slowed

<u>Prolonged Exercise</u>

- Exercise that can be sustained from 30-180 min
- **During prolonged submaximal exercise** – intensity and duration dictate energy source depletion and fatigue
    o Muscle glycogen depletion is a major source of fatigue during higher intensities; is the primary source of energy during the first 30 min
    o Fat utilization increases with longer exercise duration and during lower intensities; fat depletion is not normally a cause of fatigue
    o Blood glucose depletion is greater at higher intensities and longer duration exercise, use can decrease as fat usage increases
- Muscle and liver glycogen, fats, and glucose are all used for significant exercise durations such as a marathon; glycogen depletion is the predominant limiting factor for fatigue

Learn More: Sport Nutrition Textbook pgs 68-74

METABOLIC ADAPTATIONS TO EXERCISE TRAINING

- **Muscular adaptations to aerobic training that improve endurance capacity:**
    - Increased capillary density
    - Increased mitochondrial size and quantity
    - Increased activity of the TCA cycle and oxidative enzymes
    - Increased capacity to use fat as an energy source (spares glycogen)
    - Increased cross-sectional area of type I fibers
    - Decreased lactate accumulation
    - Increased cardiac efficiency and output and improved oxygen delivery to working muscle
    - Increased VO$_2$max
    - Attenuated stress hormone responses that deplete glycogen
- **Muscular adaptations to strength, power or speed training:**
    - Enhanced immediate ATP and PCr energy delivery systems
    - Enhanced short-term glycolytic energy delivery systems
    - Increased metabolic buffering capacity
    - Increased force and power output, muscle fiber hypertrophy
    - Improved economy

Learn More: Sport Nutrition Textbook pgs 74-75

SECTION 3 • REVIEW YOUR KNOWLEDGE

Match the Following Terms

1. _____ Sarcomere

2. _____ T-tubules

3. _____ Myoglobin

4. _____ Interleukin-6

5. _____ Actin

6. _____ Lipolysis

7. _____ ATPase

8. _____ Myosin

9. _____ TCA cycle

10. _____ Tropomyosin

a. Cytokine that stimulates glycogen breakdown

b. Transports oxygen

c. Aerobic metabolism that occurs in the mitochondrion

d. Contractile unit of a muscle fiber

e. Metabolism of fat stores

f. Thin myofilament

g. Transports action potential to sarcoplasmic reticulum

h. Enzyme that breaks down ATP for energy

i. Protein filament that blocks binding sites on actin

j. Thick myofilament

Knowledge and Competency Exercises

11. _____ muscle fibers have fast contractile speed capability with an oxidative capacity that makes them moderately resistant to fatigue.

12. Muscle fibers are recruited by size and speed in the following order: _____, then _____, and finally _____ when needed.

13. List the three primary sources of energy metabolism (modes of ATP resynthesis) in the order they occur based on activity duration.

a) _____   b) _____   c) _____

14. True or False? *(circle one)* PCr provides energy that is sufficient to fuel short duration, high-intensity exercise such as interval sprints.

15. True or False? *(circle one)* Hydrogen ions released during glycolysis lower the pH level in muscle, increasing enzyme activity.

16. List four sources of energy storage in the human body.

a) _____   b) _____   c) _____   d) _____

17. Fat stores provide fuel at a rate that can maintain exercise intensity up to _____ VO_2max.

18. Fill in the missing components of the following table addressing hormones that regulate energy metabolism.

Hormone	Source	Stimuli for Activation	Actions
Insulin	Pancreas		
Epinephrine		Stress and drop in blood glucose	
	Adrenal cortex		Stimulates protein breakdown and lipolysis
Growth Hormone		Stress	

19. True or False? *(circle one)* Glycogen depletion is the limiting factor for fatigue during prolonged, submaximal exercise.

20. List two muscular adaptations to aerobic training that improve endurance capacity.

a) _____

b) _____

• ASSESS YOUR KNOWLEDGE

SECTION 4

1. Which of the following structures function to store calcium for use during muscular contractions?

   a. Sarcomere
   b. Myosin
   c. Sarcoplasmic Reticulum
   d. Myoglobin

2. Type I muscle fibers do NOT present with which of the following characteristics?

   a. Slow contraction rate
   b. High capacity for oxidative metabolism
   c. Capability to perform repeated contractions for a long period of time
   d. Low capillary density

3. Which of the following fiber types would be found in the highest proportion in a postural muscle such as the soleus?

   a. Type I fibers
   b. Type IIa fibers
   c. Type IIx fibers
   d. Type III fibers

4. Which of the following selections is the ultimate source of energy for all muscular work?

   a. PCr
   b. ATP
   c. Glycogen
   d. Fatty acids

5. Which of the following systems of metabolism involve the breakdown of carbohydrate without the presence of oxygen to fuel high-intensity, shorter duration exercise?

   a. β-oxidation
   b. PCr hydrolysis
   c. Glycolysis
   d. Lipolysis

6. Normal resting glycogen stores are usually depleted after which of the following durations of continuous intense exercise?

    a. 30 - 45 minutes
    b. 1 - 2 hours
    c. 3.5 - 5.0 hours
    d. Glycogen stores are rarely depleted

7. Energy levels within muscle are regulated by each of the following except?

    a. Enzymatic reactions
    b. Sympathetic nervous system activity
    c. Hormonal activity
    d. Lactate synthesis

8. Which of the following hormones stimulate liver glycogen breakdown and gluconeogenesis in response to a drop in blood glucose levels?

    a. Insulin
    b. Interleukin-6
    c. Glucagon
    d. Growth hormone

9. Which of the following is the primary cause of fatigue during high-intensity exercise lasting 1 to 5 minutes?

    a. PCr depletion
    b. Fat depletion
    c. Hydrogen ion accumulation
    d. Acetyl-coA accumulation

10. Which of the following is not a muscular adaptation to aerobic training?

    a. Increased mitochondrial size and quantity
    b. Increased cross-sectional area of type I muscle fibers
    c. Increased capacity to use fat as an energy source during submaximal efforts
    d. Increased short-term glycolytic energy-delivery systems

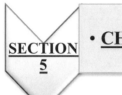

• **CHECK YOUR WORK**

SPORT NUTRITION CHAPTER 3 ANSWERS

MATCH THE FOLLOWING TERMS

1. D

2. G

3. B

4. A

5. F

6. E

7. H

8. J

9. C

10. I

KNOWLEDGE AND COMPETENCY EXERCISES

11. Type IIa

12. Type I, Type IIa, Type IIx

13. PCr hydrolysis, glycolysis, oxidative phosphorylation (aerobic metabolism)

14. True

15. False

16. **Possible answers:** Liver glycogen, muscle glycogen, blood glucose, fat, protein

17. 60%

18. See data in table.

Hormone	Source	Stimuli for Activation	Actions
Insulin	Pancreas	*Rise in glucose and amino acids*	*Glucose and amino acid uptake, inhibits lipolysis and protein breakdown*
Epinephrine	*Stress, fall in glucose*	Stress and drop in blood glucose	*Glycogen breakdown, lipolysis in adipose tissue*
Cortisol	Adrenal cortex	*Stress, hormonal activators*	Stimulates protein breakdown and lipolysis
Growth Hormone	*Anterior pituitary gland*	Stress	*Liver glycogen breakdown, lipolysis in adipose tissue, cortisol secretion*

19. True

20. **Possible choices**: increased capillary density, increased mitochondrial size and quantity, increased activity of the TCA cycle and oxidative enzymes, increased capacity to use fat as an energy source, spares glycogen, increased cross-sectional area of type I fibers, decreased lactate accumulation, increased cardiac output, VO_2max and oxygen delivery to working muscle, attenuated stress hormone responses that deplete glycogen

ASSESS YOUR KNOWLEDGE

1. C	6. B
2. D	7. D
3. A	8. C
4. B	9. C
5. C	10. D

SECTION 1 • LEARNING GOALS

Upon completing this section, along with its corresponding chapter, you should understand the following:

1. The definitions of energy, work, power, energy expenditure, calories, and joules

2. The concept of energy efficiency and its various definitions

3. The methods for measuring the energy content of food

4. The Atwater energy values for carbohydrates, fats, and proteins

5. The concept of the coefficient of digestibility for food products, and the differences in energy absorption seen between various nutrients

6. The various techniques for measuring energy expenditure including direct calorimetry, indirect calorimetry, tracer, and convenient estimate methods

7. The concept and use of the respiratory quotient during measurement of exercise energy expenditure

8. The primary components of daily energy expenditure including the resting metabolic rate (RMR), thermic effect of food (TEF), and the thermic effect of exercise (TEE)

9. Energy balance equations related to weight loss or weight gain

10. The challenges of energy balance encountered during elite-level training for specific sports

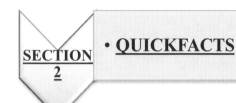

SECTION 2 • <u>QUICKFACTS</u>

DEFINING ENERGY

- **Energy** is the capacity to perform mechanical work
  - o Forms include light energy, chemical energy, heat energy, and electrical energy
- **Work = force x distance**
- **Power** is work expressed per unit of time (Power = work ÷ time)

Learn More: Sport Nutrition Textbook pg 80

QUANTIFYING ENERGY

- **Energy Expenditure (EE)** is the quantity of energy expended in metric system **kilojoules (kJ)** or English system **kilocalories (kcal)** per unit time to produce power
- **Calorie** – quantity of energy needed to raise the temperature of 1g (1ml) of water by 1 °C; due to the small unit of measurement, kilocalories are usually used
  - o 1 Kcal = 1,000 calories
  - o Example – A food product that contains 200 kcal (200,000 calories) has enough potential energy to raise the temperature of 200 L of water by 1 °C
- **Joule** – quantity of energy that can move a mass of 1g at a velocity of 1 m/s; due to the small unit of measurement, kilojoules are usually used
- **1 calorie = 4.186 J**

Learn More: Sport Nutrition Textbook pg 80

ENERGY EFFICIENCY

- **Efficiency** is expressed as the percentage of total work accomplished after energy is expended, such as during a muscular contraction

Human body is approximately 20% efficient

20% of energy produced fuels mechanical work	80% is used to maintain body temperature or wasted as excess heat

- No system is 100% efficient – Examples: gasoline engine about 20% efficient, ordinary light bulb 20% efficient, energy-saving light bulb about 80% efficient
- **Economy** – expressed as the O_2 uptake required to exercise at a given intensity
  - o Those with lower exercise economy expend more calories at a given workload due to system inefficiency – this correlates to higher perceived exertion (RPE)

Learn More: Sport Nutrition Textbook pg 81

MEASURING ENERGY CONTENT IN FOOD

- All food has energy stored within chemical bonds that is released during digestion
- **Direct calorimetry** – technique that determines the energy content of food by combustion in a device called a **bomb calorimeter** and measuring the heat that is produced
  - o Provides total energy content of food, does not provide data on digestibility or absorption

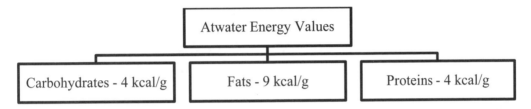

Learn More: Sport Nutrition Textbook pgs 81-82

FOOD ENERGY ABSORPTION

- **Coefficient of digestibility (COE)** – percent of food energy that is actually absorbed
  - o Example: Meal with a COE of 50 = 50% of the calories consumed would be absorbed
  - o Fiber has low COE and promotes rapid transit in the intestine while providing minimal calories
  - o Nitrogen content in protein influences COE, energy content is lost during the formation of urea

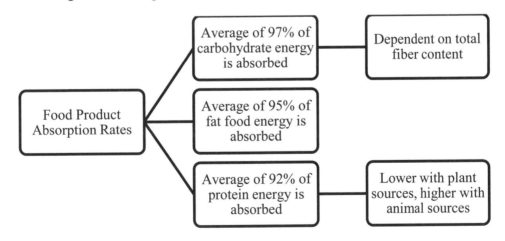

- **US Nutrient Data Bank** – content and digestibility data for over 6,000 food products

Learn More: Sport Nutrition Textbook pgs 82-83

METHODS FOR MEASURING ENERGY EXPENDITURE (EE)

- Direct Calorimetry – measurement of **heat production** to determine EE
  - **Direct Calorimetry Chamber** - uses complex chamber where heat radiated from subject is measured to determine EE, downsides include the requirement of trained personnel, specialized equipment and high cost
  - **Direct Calorimeter Suit** – used to overcome practical problems of chamber but still has limitations as it is heavy and inflexible

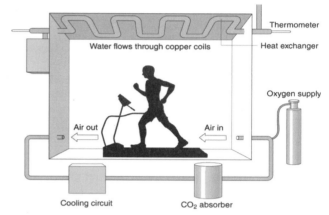

- **Indirect Calorimetry** – metabolic measurement of O_2 **uptake and** CO_2 **production** to determine EE
  - **Closed-Circuit Spirometry** – measure resting EE from respired O_2 and CO_2
  - **Open-Circuit Spirometry** – measure exercise EE from respired O_2 and CO_2
  - **Respiration Chamber** – measure EE and energy balance from O_2 and CO_2 by using specialized chamber, requires highly trained personnel and is very expensive
  - **Douglas Bag Technique** – measure EE from O_2 uptake and CO_2 production determined from analysis of expiration collected in specialized bag apparatus
  - **Breath-by-Breath Technique** – improves Douglas Bag technique by using computers and fast response O_2 and CO_2 analyzers to provide online breath-by-breath analysis
  - **Tracer Methods – Doubly Labeled Water Technique** and **Labeled Bicarbonate Technique** use ingested isotopes that reveal CO_2 production and therefore measure EE
- **Convenient Estimate Methods** – less complicated yet less accurate methods for measuring EE during natural physical activity
  - **Heart Rate Monitoring** – HR has linear relationship with O_2 uptake at submaximal exercise intensities, many limitations make it less than optimal for individual assessment
  - **Accelerometry** – estimation of EE by using accelerometer attached to the body that registers movements throughout the day; tends to underestimate energy expenditure
  - **Physical Activity Records, Activity Diaries** – rough estimation of EE based on recall data from a 24-hour period

Learn More: Sport Nutrition Textbook pgs 83-90

RESPIRATORY QUOTIENT

- **Respiratory Quotient (RQ)** – ratio of O_2 uptake and CO_2 production reveals primary substrate used and total EE
- Valid and reliable from resting state to steady state exercise up to 85% VO_2max, not above due to hyperventilation
  - RQ is close to 1.0 when carbohydrates (glucose) are used
  - RQ is close to 0.7 when fats (palmitic acid) are used

o RQ is close to 0.83 when a combination of carbohydrates and fats are used

o Varies for protein based on nitrogen and sulfur content

- Based on the premise that exchange of O_2 and CO_2 in the mouth during respiration represents the same processes that occur in active tissues to oxidize fuel

Learn More: Sport Nutrition Textbook pgs 87-88

COMPONENTS OF ENERGY EXPENDITURE

- Three primary components of daily EE:
  - **Resting Metabolic Rate (RMR)** – energy required to maintain normal resting functions, **accounts for 60% to 75% of daily EE** in relatively inactive people
    - Muscle mass accounts for 20% of the RMR
    - Organs such as the liver, gut, kidneys and heart account for 75% of the RMR
    - Adipose tissue accounts for less than 5% of the RMR
    - Influenced by age (decreases), gender (males are higher), body composition and genetics
  - **Thermic Effect of Food (TEF)** – increase in EE that occurs for up to 8 hours after ingestion of a meal (result of digestion, absorption, metabolizing and storage actions), **accounts for approximately 10% of daily EE**
    - Magnitude of TEF depends on energy content, size and composition of the meal
    - Complex carbohydrates and protein increase the TEF
  - **Thermic Effect of Exercise (TEE)** – energy required for activity, includes all EE above RMR and TEF, represents the most variable component
    - Usually accounts for 15% to 30% of daily EE but can reach up to 80% during heavy endurance training or competition

Learn More: Sport Nutrition Textbook pgs 90-92

ENERGY BALANCE AND ATHLETIC CHALLENGES

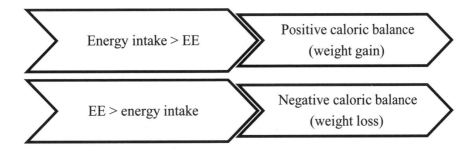

Energy intake > EE → Positive caloric balance (weight gain)

EE > energy intake → Negative caloric balance (weight loss)

- Energy balance challenges predominate in many sports where body composition is integral to success

Lower Limits

- o   Female dancers and gymnasts often have extremely low intake levels between 1,000 kcal/day and 2,000 kcal/day, in some cases this is only 1.2-1.4 times the RMR which can result in nutritional deficiencies and immune dysfunction

Upper Limits

- o   Cycling, triathlon, cross-country skiing and ultra-endurance running may require energy expenditures as high as 8,600 kcal/day (cross-country skiing), resulting in a constant challenge to consume enough food to meet energy needs
- o   Well-trained endurance athletes have been documented expending more than 1,000 kcal/hr for prolonged periods
- o   During the 3-week, 3,500 km Tour de France event, average daily energy expenditure has been measured at 6,000 kcal/day

Learn More: Sport Nutrition Textbook pgs 92-96

SECTION 3 • REVIEW YOUR KNOWLEDGE

Match the Following Terms

1. _____ Energy
2. _____ Open-circuit spirometry
3. _____ Direct calorimetry
4. _____ Coefficient of digestibility
5. _____ Nitrogen
6. _____ Calorie
7. _____ Respiratory quotient
8. _____ Joule
9. _____ Labeled bicarbonate
10. _____ Work

a. Reveals the primary substrate used during exercise

b. Energy needed to move a mass of 1g at a velocity of 1m/s

c. Method of measuring exercise energy expenditure

d. Percentage of food energy that is absorbed

e. Example of a tracer method for measuring energy expenditure

f. Represents the capacity to perform work

g. Force x Distance

h. Found in all animal protein sources

i. Measurement of heat to determine energy expenditure

j. Energy needed to raise the temperature of 1g of water by 1° C

Knowledge and Competency Exercises

11. _____ is the ratio of total work to energy expended.

12. True or False? *(circle one)* Fiber reduces the coefficient of digestibility of a meal and promotes rapid transport of digested food through the intestines.

13. Rank the following food products from highest (1) to lowest (5) in relation to their coefficient of digestibility.

_____ Egg protein   _____ Dairy fat

_____ Vegetable protein   _____ Vegetable fat

_____ Legume protein

14. Identify the caloric yield per gram consumed for the following macronutrients based on the Atwater factors.

_____ Carbohydrates   _____ Fats   _____ Proteins

15. List three methods of measuring energy expenditure through indirect calorimetry.

a) _____

b) _____

c) _____

16. If _____ was the predominant fuel source during an exercise session, the measured respiratory quotient would be around 0.7.

17. List the three primary components of energy expenditure.

a) _____   b) _____   c) _____

18. True or False? *(circle one)* The thermic effect of food can increase energy expenditure for up to 8 hours after ingestion of a meal.

19. True or False? *(circle one)* The thermic effect of exercise is normally between 15-30% but can account for up to 80% of daily energy expenditure during elite-level, heavy endurance training competitions.

20. If energy intake _____ energy expenditure, the body will be in a positive caloric balance and weight gain will occur.

• PRACTICAL APPLICATIONS

SECTION 4

CASE STUDY 1 – DIETARY REVIEW

Review the following data on Mr. Johnson's daily food intake and answer the questions that follow. The coefficient of digestibility for each meal is as follows: breakfast – 94, lunch – 89, dinner – 82, dessert – 96.

Meal	Food Product	Carbohydrate (g)	Sugar (g)	Fiber (g)	Fat (g)	Protein (g)
Breakfast	Raisin Bran	37	15	6	1	5
	1 cup of milk	29	9	0	6	5
	Coffee (creamer)	15	15	0	2	0
Lunch	Taco salad	63	17	5	61	36
	12oz Coke	39	39	0	0	0
Dinner	Meatloaf	10	5	1	30	30
	Mashed potatoes	12	3	1	1	2
	Mixed veggies	30	12	12	0	8
Dessert	Apple pie	60	45	3	18	4
	Ice cream	32	20	0	24	5

1. How many total calories did Mr. Johnson consume? _____

2. How many calories were actually absorbed? _____

3. What percentage of the calories ingested came from simple sugars? _____ (Sugar calories ÷ Total calories)

4. What percentage of the calories ingested came from fat? _____ (Fat calories ÷ Total calories)

5. What are two primary modifications that could be made to Mr. Johnson's diet that would increase the relative thermic effect of food from his diet and allow him a better chance for attaining a negative caloric balance for weight loss?

a) _____

b) _____

CASE STUDY 2 – CREEPING OBESITY

Review the data on the following table and answer the corresponding questions. The table displays the daily caloric intake and expenditure for a client during a 1-week period. Note: to gain or lose one pound of fat, an individual needs to be in a positive or negative caloric balance of 3,500 kcal.

	Mon	Tues	Wed	Thurs	Fri	Sat	Sun
INTAKE	2550 kcal	2730 kcal	2205 kcal	2640 kcal	3205 kcal	3100 kcal	2460 kcal
EXPENDITURE	2450 kcal	2305 kcal	2330 kcal	2550 kcal	2460 kcal	2720 kcal	2200 kcal

1. What was the individual's weekly caloric intake? _____

2. What was the individual's weekly caloric expenditure? _____

3. Was the individual in a positive or negative caloric balance? _____

4. Theoretically, if the individual continued with identical intake and expenditure patterns, how long would it take for him to lose or gain one pound of fat? _____

5. How much weight would he potentially lose or gain each month? _____

SECTION 5 • ASSESS YOUR KNOWLEDGE

1. Which of the following selections is defined by mechanical work expressed per unit of time?

    a. Energy
    b. Joule
    c. Power
    d. Net efficiency

2. Approximately how efficient is the human body when using energy produced during muscular contractions or other forms of mechanical work?

    a. 20% efficient
    b. 35% efficient
    c. 70% efficient
    d. 100% efficient

3. Which of the following devices can be used to directly measure the caloric content of a food product in the clinical setting?

    a. Spirometer
    b. Direct calorimetry chamber
    c. Douglas bag
    d. Bomb calorimeter

4. According to the Atwater energy values, fat provides approximately how many kilocalories per gram consumed?

    a. 2 kcal/g
    b. 4 kcal/g
    c. 7 kcal/g
    d. 9 kcal/g

5. Which of the following food products has the highest coefficient of digestibility (COE)?

    a. Plant source protein
    b. Fat
    c. Animal source protein
    d. Sugar

6. Which of the following would produce a respiratory quotient of 1.0 if it was the primary energy used during exercise?

    a. Protein
    b. Glucose
    c. Glycogen
    d. Fat

7. Which of the following selections is the greatest component of energy expenditure among sedentary individuals?

    a. Thermic effect of food (TEF)
    b. Resting metabolic rate (RMR)
    c. Thermic effect of exercise (TEE)
    d. Hormonal actions related to emotion (HAE)

8. Which of the following is incorrect as it relates to resting metabolic rate (RMR)?

    a. Greater total muscle mass increases RMR
    b. RMR increases with age
    c. Actions of organs such as the liver, kidneys and heart account for up to 75% of the RMR
    d. Genetics have a significant influence on RMR

9. Which of the following nutrients would produce the greatest thermic effect and subsequent increase in energy expenditure hours after consumption?

    a. Simple carbohydrates
    b. Lean protein
    c. Fat
    d. Alcohol

10. Well-trained endurance athletes have been documented expending calories at rates up to _____, making energy balance difficult.

    a. 300 kcal/hour
    b. 750 kcal/hour
    c. 1,000 kcal/hour
    d. 1,300 kcal/hour

SECTION 6 • CHECK YOUR WORK

SPORT NUTRITION CHAPTER 4 ANSWERS

Match the Following Terms

1. F	5. H	9. E
2. C	6. J	10. G
3. I	7. A	
4. D	8. B	

Knowledge and Competency Exercises

11. Gross efficiency

12. True

13. 1 – Egg protein, 2 -Dairy fat, 3 – Vegetable fat, 4 – Vegetable protein, 5 – Legume protein

14. 4 kcal – carbohydrates, 9 kcal – fats, 4 kcal - proteins

15. Closed-circuit spirometry, open-circuit spirometry, use of a respiration chamber, Douglas Bag technique, Breath-by-Breath technique, tracer methods

16. Fat

17. Resting metabolic rate (RMR), thermic effect of food (TEF), thermic effect of exercise (TEE)

18. True

19. True

20. Exceeds

Case Study 1

1. Breakfast: Carbohydrates – 324 kcal, Fats – 81 kcal, Protein – 40 kcal, Total kcal - 445

Lunch: Carbohydrates – 408 kcal, Fats – 549 kcal, Protein – 144 kcal, Total kcal - 1101

Dinner: Carbohydrates – 208 kcal, Fats – 279 kcal, Protein – 160 kcal, Total kcal - 647

Dessert: Carbohydrates – 368 kcal, Fats – 378 kcal, Protein – 36 kcal, Total kcal - 782

Daily Total = 2975 kcal

2. Breakfast: Total kcal considering COE – 418.3

Lunch: Total kcal considering COE - 979.9

Dinner: Total kcal considering COE - 530.5

Dessert: Total kcal considering COE - 750.7

Daily Total = 2679 kcal

3. 720/2975 = 24%

4. 1287/2975 = 43%

5. a) Reduce simple sugar intake as 25% is too high

b) Reduce fat intake as intake is too high

Case Study 2

1. 18,890 kcal

2. 17,015 kcal

3. Positive caloric balance

4. Approximately two weeks

5. Potential gain of 2 pounds of fat each month without accounting for metabolic compensations

Assess Your Knowledge

1. C	5. D	9. B
2. A	6. B	10. C
3. D	7. B	
4. D	8. B	

SECTION 1 • LEARNING GOALS

Upon completing this section, along with its corresponding chapter, you should understand the following:

1. The anatomy, primary function, and hormonal and nervous regulation of the gastrointestinal (GI) tract

2. The processes involved in carbohydrate, fat and protein digestion

3. The processes involved in carbohydrate, fat, protein, water, vitamin and mineral absorption

4. The functions of natural bacteria in the colon and the potential benefits of probiotics

5. The factors that have an effect on the rate of gastric emptying

6. Potential GI problems encountered during and after exercise

7. The primary physiological, mechanical, and nutritional causes and general guidelines for reducing the risk of exercise-related GI problems

SECTION 2 • <u>QUICKFACTS</u>

THE GASTROINTESTINAL (GI) TRACT

- Functions to provide the body with nutrients, water, and electrolytes from ingested food
- Is a 6m to 8m long tubular structure reaching from the mouth to the anus where food is processed for 1-3 days prior to the elimination of the end product
- **Transit time** – time spent in a specific section of the tract (e.g. 3 to 10 hours in the small intestine)
- **Digestion** – processes involved in the breakdown of food into small units for absorption
- **Absorption** – processes involved in transporting nutrients from the small intestine to the blood or lymph system

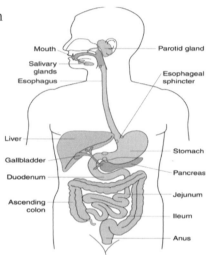

    Learn More: Sport Nutrition Textbook pgs 100 & 103

ANATOMY AND FUNCTION OF THE GI TRACT

- **Mouth** – provides for mechanical digestion via mastication (chewing)
  - Mastication serves three purposes:
    1. Reduces the size of food particles
    2. Increases the surface area (SA) of food to increase the contact area for digestive enzymes
    3. Mixes food particles with saliva and digestive enzymes
- **Salivary glands** – parotid, sublingual, and submandibular glands in the mouth release enzymes to break down food and protect from oral bacteria
- **Esophagus** – transports food to stomach via rhythmical patterns of contraction and relaxation
  - Esophageal sphincter dysfunction causes acid reflux (heartburn)
- **Stomach** – structure that stores around 1.5 L of food and fluid, can stretch to hold up to 6.0 L
  - Primary functions:
    1. Store large quantities of food until it can be accommodated into the intestine
    2. Mix food with gastric secretions and hydrochloric (HCl) acid to break down proteins and form a homogenous, acidic, soup-like liquid called **chyme**
    3. Regulate the emptying of chyme into the small intestine via the pyloric sphincter

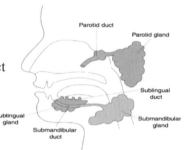

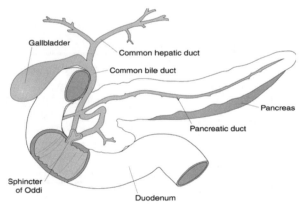

- **Pancreas** – secretes digestive enzymes and sodium bicarbonate to buffer the acidity of chyme
- **Liver** – secretes bile acids to facilitate the digestion and absorption of fats
- **Gallbladder** – provides temporary storage and increases the concentration of bile
- **Small intestine** (SI) – divided into the duodenum, jejunum, and ileum; provides for **95%** of all water, nutrient and electrolyte absorption
  - High absorption capability is due to the following structures of the intestinal wall lining that collectively creates a surface area larger than a tennis court:
    1. **Folds of Kerking**
    2. Finger-like projections in the intestinal wall lining called **villi**
    3. Numerous **microvilli** that create a **brush border** on the villi
  - Enhances absorption rate 600x greater than a flat tube lining
- **Large intestine** – divided into the colon, rectum, and anal canal (colon is further divided into ascending, transverse, descending, and sigmoid sections); provides additional absorption of electrolytes and stores feces until they can be expelled

Learn More: Sport Nutrition Textbook pgs 100-104

REGULATION OF THE GI TRACT
- Neuroendocrine controls of the GI tract:
  1. The autonomic nervous system (ANS) regulates **motility** (movement of food)
     - Vagus nerve provides ANS regulation for the esophagus, stomach, pancreas, gallbladder, small intestine, and upper section of large intestine
  2. Special sensory neurons not associated with the ANS in the actual GI tract wall regulate actions
  3. Hormones released by endocrine and paracrine glands regulate actions

Primary regulatory hormones of the GI tract:

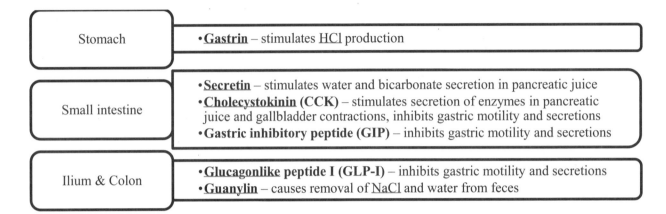

Stomach	•**Gastrin** – stimulates <u>HCl</u> production
Small intestine	•**Secretin** – stimulates water and bicarbonate secretion in pancreatic juice •**Cholecystokinin (CCK)** – stimulates secretion of enzymes in pancreatic juice and gallbladder contractions, inhibits gastric motility and secretions •**Gastric inhibitory peptide (GIP)** – inhibits gastric motility and secretions
Ilium & Colon	•**Glucagonlike peptide I (GLP-I)** – inhibits gastric motility and secretions •**Guanylin** – causes removal of <u>NaCl</u> and water from feces

Learn More: Sport Nutrition Textbook pgs 104-105

NUTRIENT DIGESTION

- Digestion starts as soon as food enters the mouth and may take 4-6 hours to complete; various specific enzymes are used to digest each type of macronutrient
- **Carbohydrate digestion** – initiated by salivary enzymes that break down starches into simple sugars (Ex: prolonged chewing of a cracker causes increased sweetness), usually 30%-40% digested when leaving the stomach; in the small intestine metabolism increases to break nutrients into smaller units for proper absorption
  - Digestive dysfunction occurs when enzymes in the small intestine cannot metabolize a specific saccharide (e.g., lactose intolerance occurs with lactase dysfunction)
  - Fiber (cellulose) resists enzymatic breakdown; bacteria in the large intestine can provide for fermentation for minimal metabolism (same process as yeast fermenting sugar in grape juice to produce wine)
    - Fermentation produces hydrogen, CO_2, volatile fatty acids (FA), and methane gas – excessive fiber intake increases the risk for GI distress
- **Fat digestion** – initiated by salivary enzyme lingual lipase which splits triglycerides into FAs and glycerol; enzymes in the stomach further digest short-chain and medium-chain FAs; enzymes in the small intestine further digest long-chain FAs; bile also plays a major role in metabolism as fats enter the intestine
- **Protein digestion** – initiated in the stomach with HCl acid, continued by enzymes in the small intestine which break down polypeptides into simple amino acids

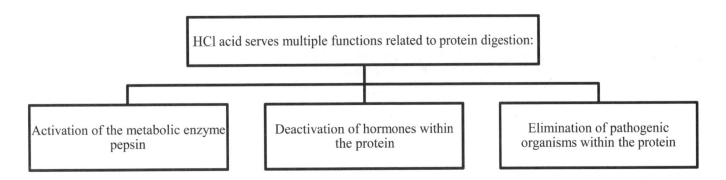

- A comprehensive overview of digestive enzymes and their functions can be reviewed in Table 5.3 on page 106

Learn More: Sport Nutrition Textbook pgs 104-109

NUTRIENT ABSORPTION

- Most absorption occurs at the epithelial cells of the small intestine via one of three modes;

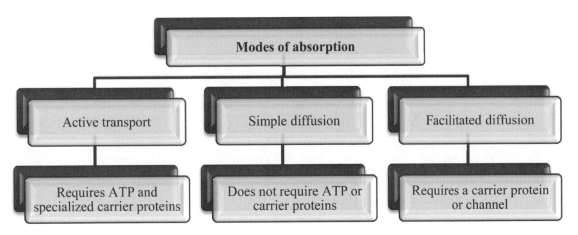

Macronutrients then enter circulation via the hepatic portal vein for delivery to the liver

- o Fats can also enter circulation via the lymphatic system and the subclavian veins

- **Carbohydrate absorption** – monosaccharides are transported by special carriers across epithelial cells of the small intestine
- **Fat absorption** – FAs are transported by special carriers called micelles (derived from bile salts) and diffused across epithelial cells of the small intestine; presence of bile allows high absorption (97%), while absence allows low absorption (50%)
- **Protein absorption** – amino acids and peptides are absorbed by carrier-mediated active transport across epithelial cells of the small intestine
- **Water absorption** – 99% of absorption takes place in the small intestine via simple diffusion

- **Vitamin absorption** – occurs in the small intestine; fat-soluble vitamins are absorbed with FAs through facilitated diffusion, water-soluble vitamins are absorbed with water through simple diffusion
- **Mineral absorption** – not efficiently absorbed in intestines allowing intake in food to be much higher than actual requirements; absorbed at differing rates based on chemical form ingested. (Example – heme iron has ~15% absorption rate, non-heme iron has 2-10% absorption rate)

Learn More: Sport Nutrition Textbook pgs 109-113

GI BACTERIA

- The large intestine contains about 1 kg of various bacteria, while in healthy people the stomach and small intestine have relatively small quantities due to gastric acid
- Quantity and type of bacteria found in the GI tract can vary greatly based on health, diet and age and is actually sterile at birth
- Bacteria in the large intestine:
  - Digest carbohydrates (fiber), proteins, and fats that escape absorption in the small intestine
  - Help produce vitamin K and various B vitamins (Bacterial vitamin K production is important because intake in food is generally insufficient)

Learn More: Sport Nutrition Textbook pgs 113-114

PROBIOTICS AND PREBIOTICS

- Beneficial bacteria or yeasts marketed as a supplement or found in certain foods such as yogurt; the most common form is the lactic acid bacteria strains
- Probiotics lower "bad or infectious bacteria" and increase "good bacteria" in the colon
- Prebiotics – foods that good bacteria in the colon feed on that stimulate their growth (e.g., wheat, bananas, oats, onions)
- Research-based claims related to probiotics:
  - Can treat and prevent acute diarrhea and antibiotic-induced diarrhea
  - Lower pH in the colon to create a less suitable environment for infectious bacteria
  - Enhance immune function
  - May reduce the severity of colds, respiratory conditions, and allergies
- Additional purported claims:
  - Combat the negative effects of excessive alcohol intake, stress, exposure to toxic substances, and other diseases

Learn More: Sport Nutrition Textbook pg 114

REGULATION OF GASTRIC EMPTYING

- Food generally takes 1 to 4 hrs to leave the stomach depending on meal content
- Emptying is initiated by contraction of pacemaker cells in the stomach wall that push chyme through the pyloric sphincter into the small intestine
- Contractions and emptying are controlled by nervous and/or hormonal signals

<u>Factors that can affect gastric emptying:</u>

1. **Smell, sight, or thought of food** – gastrin is released which speeds emptying
2. **Volume of food or drink ingested** – increased volume speeds emptying, particularly during full stomach wall extension
3. **Energy density of food or drink ingested** – increased energy density slows emptying
4. **Temperature of food or drink ingested** – very hot or cold drinks may slow emptying
5. **Osmolarity of food or drink ingested** – increased osmolarity (quantity of dissolvable particles in fluid) slows emptying and decreases water absorption
6. **Body temperature and dehydration** – hyperthermia and dehydration may slow emptying
7. **Type and intensity of exercise** – exercise intensity above 80% of VO_2max and/or intermittent high-intensity exercise (e.g., interval sprinting) slows emptying
8. **Gender** – women have slower emptying rates which is believed to be a contributing factor of frequent prolonged-exercise GI complaints
9. **Psychological stress and anxiety** – both slow emptying due to hormonal actions which reduce blood flow to the GI tract

Learn More: Sport Nutrition Textbook pgs 114-116

EXERCISE RELATED GI PROBLEMS

- 30%-50% of endurance athletes experience GI issues related to their training
- GI issues seem to occur more frequently:
  - Among young women
  - During running or other high-impact activities when compared to cycling or swimming

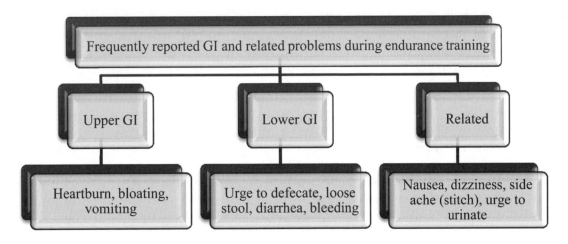

Learn More: Sport Nutrition Textbook pgs 116-117

CAUSES OF EXERCISE-RELATED GI PROBLEMS

- **Potential physiological causes**
  - Anxiety
  - Significantly reduced blood flow to the GI tract
    - Severe cases can result in damage to the large intestine
- **Potential mechanical causes**
  - High-impact activity can potentially cause intestinal bleeding and blood in the feces
  - Continuous gastric jostling is thought to contribute to flatulence, diarrhea and urgency to defecate
  - Postural modification can cause increased pressure of abdomen and GI tract
  - "Swallowing" of air can cause moderate stomach distress
- **Potential nutritional causes**
  - Ingestion of fiber, fat, protein or fructose during or immediately prior to training
  - Dehydration can exacerbate GI symptoms
  - Ingestion of fluid with high osmolarities (>500mOsm/L)
  - Ingestion of dairy products

Learn More: Sport Nutrition Textbook pgs 117-118

PREVENTION OF EXERCISE-RELATED GI PROBLEMS

- Research-based guidelines for preventing GI problems are limited, but the following recommendations are purported to reduce risk:
  - **Avoid milk products** – even mild lactose intolerance can cause problems during exercise
  - **Avoid high-fiber foods** – increased bowel movement and GI discomfort may occur if ingested prior to competition
  - **Avoid aspirin and NSAIDs** – increase the incidence of GI complaints
  - **Avoid high-fructose foods and drinks** – not rapidly absorbed and known to be less tolerated than high-glucose selections
  - **Avoid dehydration** – can exacerbate GI symptoms
  - **Practice new nutrition strategies** – varying strategies may meet specific needs

Learn More: Sport Nutrition Textbook pgs 118-119

SECTION 3 • <u>**REVIEW YOUR KNOWLEDGE**</u>

<u>Match the Following Terms</u>

1. _____ Salivary glands

2. _____ Secretin

3. _____ Esophageal sphincter

4. _____ Large intestine

5. _____ Motility

6. _____ Probiotics

7. _____ Liver

8. _____ Active Transport

9. _____ Gallbladder

10. ____ Villi

a. Finger-like projections in the small intestine

b. Stores feces until they can be expelled

c. Stores bile

d. Dysfunction can cause heartburn

e. Processes nutrients that are sent from the intestines

f. Release enzymes and protect against oral bacteria

g. Mode of absorption

h. Refers to the movement of food in the GI tract

i. Stimulates bicarbonate secretion in pancreatic juice

j. Beneficial bacteria that can be found in yogurt

<u>Knowledge and Competency Exercises</u>

11. The GI tract is a _____ long tubular structure that reaches from the mouth to the anus.

12. List the three primary digestive functions of the stomach.

a) _____

b) _____

c) _____

13. True or False? *(circle one)* The folds of Kirkmoore, villi and microvilli in the large intestine all function to increase surface area for optimal absorption of nutrients.

14. Fill in the following table covering the effects of GI hormones.

Hormone	Secreted by	Effect
Gastrin	Stomach	
	Small intestine	Inhibits gastric motility and secretion
Glucagonlike peptide I (GLP-I)	Ileum and colon	
Secretin		Stimulates water and bicarbonate secretion in pancreatic juice
Cholecystokinin (CCK)		Stimulates secretion of enzymes and inhibits gastric motility
Guanylin	Ileum and colon	

15. True or False? *(circle one)* Prolonged chewing of a single cracker causes it to taste sweeter because salivary enzymes break down starches and complex carbohydrates into simple sugars.

16. List three effects that HCl acid has on protein in the stomach.

a) _____

b) _____

c) _____

17. _____ requires energy in the form of ATP to facilitate absorption of nutrients.

18. True or False? *(circle one)* Fatty acids can enter circulation through the lymphatic system, the subclavian veins and the hepatic portal vein to be transported to the liver.

19. True or False? *(circle one)* The large intestine contains about 1kg of various bacteria, while the stomach and small intestines have much lower quantities due to gastric acid.

20. List five specific factors that can affect the rate of gastric emptying.

a) _____

b) _____

c) _____

d) _____

e) _____

SECTION 4 • **ASSESS YOUR KNOWLEDGE**

1. Which of the following components of the GI tract secretes sodium bicarbonate to buffer the acidity of digested food released from the stomach?

   a. Liver
   b. Pancreas
   c. Small intestine
   d. Gallbladder

2. Which of the following components of the GI tract provides for approximately 95% of all nutrient absorption?

   a. Stomach
   b. Liver
   c. Large intestine
   d. Small intestine

3. Which of the following hormones is secreted in the stomach to stimulate hydrochloric (HCl) acid production for the breakdown of nutrients and elimination of bacteria?

   a. Secretin
   b. Guanylin
   c. Gastrin
   d. Cholecystokinin (CCK)

4. Which of the following nutrients is digested in the large intestine by a process called fermentation?

   a. Fat
   b. Fiber
   c. Vegetable protein
   d. Minerals

5. The absence of bile will significantly reduce the absorption rate of which of the following nutrients?

   a. Fat
   b. Water-soluble vitamins
   c. Protein
   d. Monosaccharides

6. Probiotics have been suggested to provide which of the following benefits?

   a. Increased protein synthesis during most types of high-stress training
   b. Reduction in the risk of intestinal bleeding during endurance training
   c. Prevention of acute or antibiotic-induced diarrhea
   d. Reduction in the risk of upper GI symptoms during endurance training

7. Which of the following statements associated with factors that can affect the rate of gastric emptying is INCORRECT?

   a. Gastrin is released during the smell, sight or thought of food, causing an increase in gastric emptying
   b. Increased energy density and/or osmolarity of an ingested beverage increases the rate of gastric emptying
   c. Stress and anxiety decrease the rate of gastric emptying
   d. Exercise intensity above 80% of the VO_2max decreases the rate of gastric emptying

8. Which of the following is not a common lower GI symptom during prolonged endurance training?

   a. Intestinal bleeding
   b. Loose stool
   c. Heartburn
   d. Diarrhea

9. Which of the following is not a major mechanical cause of exercise-related GI problems?

   a. Continual impacts
   b. Gastric jostling
   c. Posture
   d. Dehydration

10. Which of the following is not a valid guideline for preventing exercise-related GI problems?

   a. Avoid milk products during exercise
   b. Avoid high-fiber foods the day of competition for an endurance event
   c. Avoid aspirin and NSAIDs during prolonged exercise
   d. Avoid beverages that contain primarily glucose as the carbohydrate source

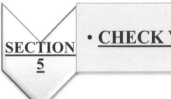

SPORT NUTRITION CHAPTER 5 ANSWERS

Match the Following Terms

1. F   6. J

2. I   7. E

3. D   8. G

4. B   9. C

5. H   10. A

Knowledge and Competency Exercises

11. 6m to 8m

12. **a)** Stores large quantities of food until it can be accommodated into the intestine **b)** Mixes food with gastric secretions and hydrochloric (HCl) acid to break down proteins and form a homogenous, acidic, soup-like liquid or paste called chyme **c)** Regulates emptying of chyme into the small intestine by action of the pyloric sphincter

13. False

14.

Hormone	Secreted by	Effect
Gastrin	Stomach	*Stimulates HCl production, stimulates secretion of pepsinogen*
Gastric inhibitory peptide (GIP)	Small intestine	Inhibits gastric motility and secretion
Glucagonlike peptide I (GLP-I)	*Ileum and colon*	*Inhibits gastric motility and secretion*
Secretin	*Small intestine*	Stimulates water and bicarbonate secretion in pancreatic juice
Cholecystokinin (CCK)	*Small intestine*	Stimulates secretion of enzymes and inhibits gastric motility
Guanylin	Ileum and colon	*Causes removal of NaCl and water from feces*

15. True

16. **a)** Activates the metabolic enzyme pepsin, **b)** deactivates hormones within the protein, and **c)** kills pathogenic organisms within the protein

17. Active transport

18. True

19. True

20. **Potential factors that can affect gastric emptying:** Smell, sight, or thought of food, volume of food or drink ingested, energy density of food or drink ingested, temperature of food or drink ingested, osmolarity of food or drink ingested, body temperature and dehydration, type and intensity of exercise, gender, psychological stress and anxiety

Assess Your Knowledge

1. B

2. D

3. C

4. B

5. A

6. C

7. B

8. C

9. D

10. D

SECTION 1 • LEARNING GOALS

Upon completing this section, along with its corresponding chapter, you should understand the following:

1. How proper carbohydrate (CHO) intake positively affects performance measures

2. The storage forms of CHO within the human body

3. The mechanisms by which blood glucose is stabilized at rest and during exercise

4. The causes, symptoms, and remedy for acute or prolonged hypoglycemia

5. The recommendations for CHO intake that allow an athlete to restore glycogen on a daily basis

6. The concepts of glycemic index and glycemic load

7. The concepts and optimal strategies related to CHO intake in specified timeframes before (days, hours, minutes), during, and after competition or exercise

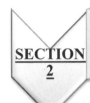

RECOGNIZING CARBOHYDRATES FOR PERFORMANCE
- 100 years ago beef was considered the most important component of an athlete's diet
- Current knowledge illustrates that carbohydrates (CHO) are necessary for optimal performance during intermittent high-intensity training, prolonged training, and cognitive/motor skill execution
- Most research over the last 30 years has focused on:
    - Proper CHO intake prior to competition or intense training to increase muscle and liver glycogen reserves for prolonged performance
    - Proper CHO intake during competition or training that reduces the risk for hypoglycemia
    - Proper CHO intake after competition or training for optimal recovery

Learn More: Sport Nutrition Textbook pg 122

HISTORY OF CARBOHYDRATE INTAKE RESEARCH
- Specific developing research examples that led to current CHO intake recommendations:
    - Krogh and Lindhart (1920) compared exercise performance using either a high-fat (bacon, butter, eggs, cream, and cabbage) or a high-CHO (potatoes, flour, bread, cake, marmalade, and sugar) diet for three days; the high-fat group experienced significant fatigue by the exercise protocol while the high-CHO group did not
    - Levine, Gordon, and Derick (1924) examined participants of the Boston Marathon and found that individuals who consumed CHOs during the event, and followed a high-CHO diet prior to competition did not become hypoglycemic and had improved running performance
    - Dill, Edward, and Talbott (1932) compared running performance and time to exhaustion among dogs on either a high-CHO or non-CHO diet; the high-CHO diet allowed for 17-23 hours of running while the diet lacking CHOs allowed for only 4-6 hours of running
    - Christensen (1932) and Bergstrom et al (1966, 1967) showed that with increasing exercise intensity, the proportion of CHOs utilized increased; these studies indicated the critical role of muscle glycogen for performance and led to the recommendations for CHO loading prior to competition
    - Costill et al. (1973) and Coyle et al. (1984, 1986) investigated the effects of CHO feeding during exercise and the positive effects on performance and metabolism

Learn More: Sport Nutrition Textbook pgs 122-123

CARBOHYDRATE STORAGE

- Function of CHO is to provide energy for working muscle
- **Muscle glycogen** – serves as the rapid energy source for working muscle
  - Human storage is approximately 300g-400g
  - Most important energy substrate during high-intensity training
- **Liver glycogen** – serves to maintain a constant blood glucose level
  - Approximately 80g-110g available in this form (~25% total storage)
  - Liver breaks down glycogen stores **(glycogenolysis)** to release glucose; new glucose is synthesized through a process called **gluconeogenesis** to be released into circulation
    - The liver can use lactate, glycerol, pyruvate, and amino acids to produce glucose
  - **During resting conditions** – 60% of liver glucose output occurs via glycogenolysis while 40% comes from gluconeogenesis
  - **During exercise** – over 90% comes from glycogenolysis
  - Liver storage can be reduced to low levels (<20g) after overnight fast due to CHO needed by the brain

Learn More: Sport Nutrition Textbook pgs 123-124, 126

CIRCULATING BLOOD – THE GLUCOSE RESERVOIR

- Blood in circulation can be regarded as a glucose reservoir from which various tissues and muscle can tap into during rest or exercise as needed
- Glucose level in circulation is maintained close to 1g/L of blood (4.0 to 4.5mmol/L)
- **When blood glucose drops** – liver releases glucose into circulation
- **When demand for glucose drops** – liver produces less glucose or may take up glucose from circulation through the hepatic portal vein

- **When blood glucose significantly increases** (such as after a meal) – liver uses the extra CHO content to synthesize glycogen

Learn More: Sport Nutrition Textbook pgs 125

HORMONAL REGULATION OF BLOOD GLUCOSE

- **Insulin** – increases uptake and storage of glucose into various tissues
- **Glucagon** – stimulates breakdown of liver glycogen and release of glucose into circulation
- **Catecholamines (epinephrine, norepinephrine, and dopamine)** – reduce the secretion of insulin from the pancreas
- **Growth hormone**, **cortisol**, and **somatostatin** also have an effect on glucose concentration

Learn More: Sport Nutrition Textbook pg 126

HYPOGLYCEMIA

- Occurs when glucose concentrations drop below a critical level (often 3mmol/L) where the metabolic demands of the brain are not met, treated by simply ingesting CHO
- Research shows that glycogen levels are very difficult to maintain with intense training (≥3 hours per day) on consecutive days without significantly increasing CHO intake
- Increasing CHO intake from the U.S. RDA equivalent of 5-6g/kg of body weight (BW) to 10-13g/kg of BW is recommended to reduce hypoglycemia risk during intense training periods

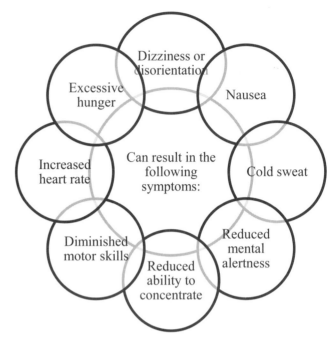

Learn More: Sport Nutrition Textbook pgs 126-127

RECOMMENDATIONS FOR CARBOHYDRATE INTAKE

- The following CHO intake recommendations developed by the International Olympic Committee (IOC) should allow an athlete to restore glycogen on a daily basis (they should be tailored to individual needs):
  - Consume 5g-12g/kg of BW each day depending on exercise intensity and duration
  - Choose moderate to **high-glycemic index** (GI) CHOs for the majority of immediate recovery meals (within 1-2 hours)
  - Consume a CHO-rich sports drink within the first hour after exercise when the appetite is suppressed
  - Recovery meals should also incorporate foods that provide some protein to promote additional glycogen restoration
  - When training sessions are spaced less than 8 hours apart, begin CHO intake as quickly as possible; a series of snacks can help to meet demand
  - During longer recovery periods (24 hours), the athlete should organize the pattern and timing of CHO-rich foods according to what is practical and comfortable based on the situation
  - Adequate total daily energy intake must be attained

Learn More: Sport Nutrition Textbook pg 128

GLYCEMIC INDEX AND GLYCEMIC LOAD

- GI refers to the increase in blood glucose and insulin in response to a standard amount of food
  - Usually based on the ingestion of 50g of CHO and subsequent measurements of blood glucose over a 2-hour period
  - A greater GI value indicates rapid absorption and delivery into circulation

o   White bread is considered a reference food with a GI value of 100

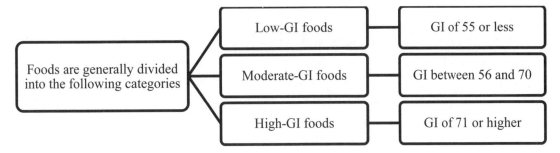

- **Glycemic load** (GL) takes the GI value for a specific food and multiplies it by the actual amount of CHO in a common serving
- GL can provide a more complete picture of the glycemic response associated with a food product than GI alone

Learn More: Sport Nutrition Textbook pg 135

CARBOHYDRATE INTAKE DAYS BEFORE COMPETITION
- When additional CHO intake is warranted, the goal is to replenish and maximize muscle glycogen stores
- **Proper carbohydrate loading** – increases time to exhaustion (endurance capacity) by an average of 20% and reduces time to complete a task (time trial, endurance performance) by 2% to 3%
  - o   Duration of exercise must be ≥90 min before performance benefits are tangible
  - o   Has no effect on sprint performance or high-intensity exercise up to 30 min

Learn More: Sport Nutrition Textbook pgs 132-133

METHODS FOR CARBOHYDRATE LOADING
- **Classical supercompensation method** – results in extremely high muscle glycogen
- **Step 1** – Engage in a glycogen-depleting bout of exercise 7 days before competition
- **Step 2** – Follow with 3 days on a high-protein, high-fat diet (6 to 4 days before competition)
- **Step 3** – Engage in another exhausting bout of exercise 4 days before competition
- **Step 4** – Follow with a very high-CHO diet for the last three days before competition
- The period of CHO deprivation with 2 bouts of exhaustive exercise stimulates increased glycogen resynthesis during the period of high-CHO intake the 3 days before competition
- Potential disadvantages:
  - o   Hypoglycemia during the low-CHO period

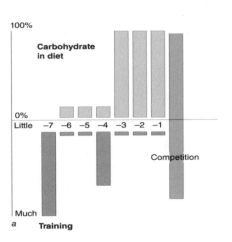

- o Practical problems such as preparation of an extreme diet
- o Gastrointestinal problems (diarrhea during high-protein, high-fat diet)
- o Poor recovery when no CHO is ingested
- o Tenseness and anxiety from a week without training (negative mental preparation)
- o Increased risk of injury
- o Mood disturbances and lethargy during the low-CHO period
- **Moderate supercompensation method** – results in nearly the same muscle glycogen storage without all of the disadvantages
  - o Slowly reduce training over a 6-day period before competition with complete rest on the last day
  - o During the same 6-day period before competition progressively increase CHO in the diet from 50% to 70% of total calories consumed

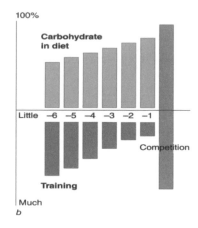

Learn More: Sport Nutrition Textbook pgs 131-132

CARBOHYDRATE INTAKE HOURS BEFORE EXERCISE

- Goal of intake is optimization of liver glycogen stores
- Recommended – ingest approximately 140g to 330g of CHO in a meal 3 to 5 hours before exercise to increase glycogen levels and improve performance
- Some of the CHO will restore muscle glycogen, but the majority is used to replenish/increase liver stores; especially important after an overnight fast

Learn More: Sport Nutrition Textbook pgs 133-134

CARBOHYDRATE INTAKE 30 TO 60 MINTUES BEFORE EXERCISE

- CHO ingestion in the hour before exercise results in a large rise in plasma glucose and insulin; with the onset of exercise this can cause **reactive hypoglycemia**

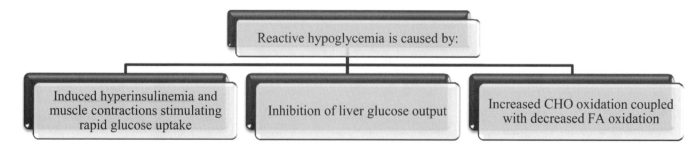

- Strategies for minimizing hypoglycemia have been investigated (i.e., ingestion of lower GI CHO food sources, fats, and/or proteins and varying the CHO load) but appear to provide no advantage
- Despite these reactions, the majority of research suggests that reactive hypoglycemia has limited effects on exercise performance

- Some athletes may be more prone to hypoglycemia, so timing of pre-exercise CHO should be based on experience
- If CHO is also ingested during exercise the potential adverse effects seem to be completely negated

Learn More: Sport Nutrition Textbook pg 134-136

CARBOHYDRATE INTAKE DURING EXERCISE

- Ingestion of 70g of CHO every hour (1.2 g/min) appears optimal for improving endurance capacity and exercise performance during exercise ≥45 min

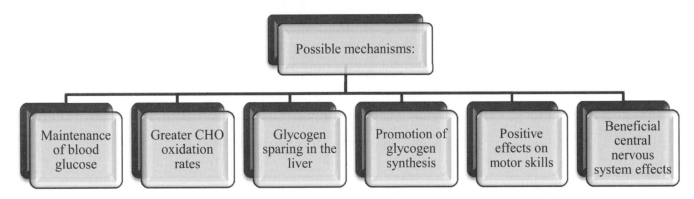

Learn More: Sport Nutrition Textbook pg 136-137

STRATEGIES TO IMPROVE USE OF CARBOHYDRATES INGESTED DURING EXERCISE

- Use of **exogenous CHO** (ingested) during exercise depends on multiple factors:
  - During the first 75 to 90 min of exercise exogenous CHO oxidation rises as CHO is emptied from the stomach; after 90 min use levels off
  - Increased exercise intensity causes increased use of exogenous CHOs
  - Greater quantity increases CHO use but overconsumption limits gastric emptying
  - Many CHOs commonly found in sports beverages can be oxidized during exercise, but research has shown that combining multiple sources can increase the rate of use (because multiple transporters can function simultaneously) while reducing the risk for digestive discomfort
    - **Rapidly oxidized CHO examples** – glucose, sucrose, maltose, maltodextrins
    - **Slowly oxidized CHO examples** – fructose, galactose, amylose
- Potential sources with the optimal quantity and type of CHO, when ingested every hour during prolonged exercise:
  - ✓ 1 L of a well-designed sports drinks (Gatorade, PowerAde)
  - ✓ 600 ml cola drink, preferably de-carbonated (flat)
  - ✓ 1.5 Power bars or Gatorade energy bars
  - ✓ 3 medium bananas
  - ✓ Approximately 3 energy gels (typically 25g CHO each)

Learn More: Sport Nutrition Textbook pgs 137-139, 141

LIMITATIONS TO INGESTED CARBOHYDRATE USE DURING EXERCISE

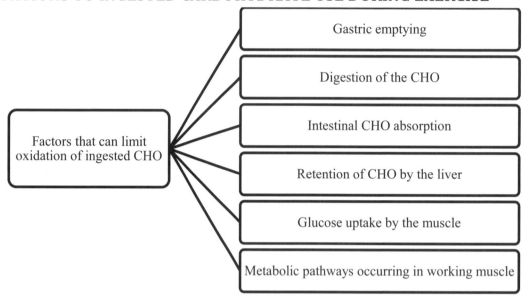

Learn More: Sport Nutrition Textbook pgs 140-141

POST-EXERCISE GLYCOGEN SYNTHESIS
- Rate of glycogen synthesis depends on:
  - The availability of glucose
  - The transport of glucose into cells, which in turn depends on:
    - Prior exercise – exercise stimulates glucose uptake for 1-2 hours post-exercise and increases insulin sensitivity
    - Insulin concentration – high insulin stimulates glucose uptake
    - Muscle glycogen content – low muscle glycogen stimulates glucose uptake
  - The activity of enzymes such as glycogen synthase
- Glycogen synthesis can occur rapidly for the first 1-2 hours after exercise (insulin-independent phase), then at a slower rate for hours after (insulin-dependent phase)

Learn More: Sport Nutrition Textbook pgs 142-144

POST-EXERCISE CARBOHYDRATE INTAKE FOR MAXIMAL GLYCOGEN RESTORATION
- Goal is to replenish depleted liver and muscle glycogen stores
- Important factors for promoting maximal muscle glycogen restoration:
  - **Timing of CHO intake** – immediate intake optimizes glycogen synthesis
  - **Rate of CHO ingestion** – ingesting higher quantities can optimize synthesis
  - **Type of CHO ingested** – high glycemic indexed CHOs are optimal for glycogen synthesis, especially immediately after exercise
  - **Ingestion of protein with CHO after exercise** – small quantity of amino acids can assist absorption of CHO (3:1 ratio of CHO:Protein)

o **Intake of caffeine** – intake during exercise increases glucose delivery to working muscle; it is thought to do the same following exercise to optimize glycogen synthesis

Learn More: Sport Nutrition Textbook pgs 144-146

POST-EXERCISE CARBOHYDRATE INTAKE SUMMARY

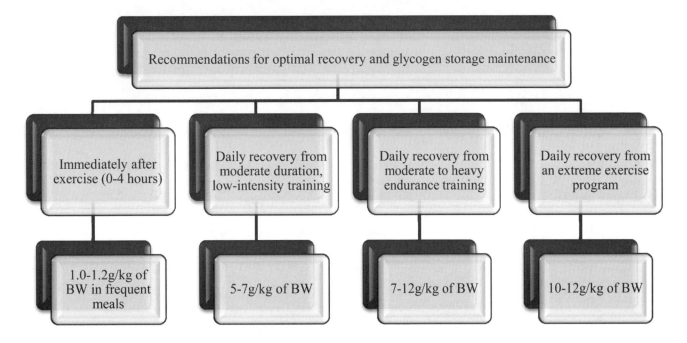

Learn More: Sport Nutrition Textbook pg 128

• REVIEW YOUR KNOWLEDGE

Match the Following Terms

1. _____ Muscle glycogen   a. Production of new glucose by the liver

2. _____ Glycemic index   b. Can result in dizziness, cold sweat, and increased heart rate

3. _____ Insulin   c. High value for a food indicates rapid absorption of CHO

4. _____ Fructose   d. Breakdown of glycogen stores

5. _____ Gluconeogenesis   e. Induced by CHO ingestion within 1 hour prior to exercise

6. _____ Glucagon   f. Hormone that stimulates the breakdown of liver glycogen

7. _____ Reactive hypoglycemia   g. Examines the insulin response to total CHO content in food

8. _____ Glycemic load   h. Readily available energy source for working muscle

9. _____ Hypoglycemia   i. Example of a slowly oxidized CHO

10. ____ Glycogenolysis   j. Increases uptake of glucose into working tissues

Knowledge and Competency Exercises

11. List three sources from which the liver can produce new glucose.

a) _____

b) _____

c) _____

12. True or False? *(circle one)* Liver glycogen storage can be reduced to very low levels (<20g) after an overnight fast.

13. Normal glucose levels in circulation are maintained close to _____ per liter of blood.

14. _____occurs when the metabolic demands of the brain cannot be maintained.

15. List three recommendations/strategies developed by the IOC related to CHO intake that should allow an athlete to restore glycogen on a daily basis.

a) _____

b) _____

c) _____

16. Provide a specific example for each of the following.

a) Low-GI food: _____

b) Moderate-GI food: _____

c) High-GI food: _____

17. Proper CHO loading has been shown to increase time to exhaustion by an average of _____, but the duration of exercise must be _____ before performance benefits are tangible.

18. List three possible mechanisms by which CHO ingestion during an exercise bout lasting 45 minutes or longer can improve endurance capacity and performance.

a) _____

b) _____

c) _____

19. True or False? *(circle one)* Research has shown that combining multiple CHO sources in a single feeding can increase the rate of energy absorption as well as reduce the risk for digestive discomfort.

20. List two food sources that could be ingested every hour during prolonged exercise to provide the appropriate quantity and type of CHO for optimum performance.

a) _____   b) _____

SECTION 4   • ASSESS YOUR KNOWLEDGE

1. Which of the following actions in the liver provides for approximately 90% of storage CHO energy use during exercise?

   a. Lipolysis
   b. Gluconeogenesis
   c. Free amino acid degradation
   d. Glycogenolysis

2. Which of the following statements related to blood glucose maintenance after ingestion of a meal is true?

   a. The liver will respond by releasing glucose into circulation
   b. The liver will respond by initiating the process of glycogenolysis
   c. The liver will use the CHO content released into circulation to synthesize glycogen if needed
   d. The kidneys will respond by releasing glucagon

3. Which of the following is not a common symptom of hypoglycemia?

   a. Nausea
   b. Flushing of the skin
   c. Excessive hunger
   d. Increased heart rate

4. Which of the following recommendations related to CHO ingestion and recovery is INCORRECT?

   a. 3.0g-3.2g/kg of BW should be ingested in frequent meals immediately after exercise (0-4 hours)
   b. 5-7g/kg of BW should be ingested for optimal daily recovery from moderate duration, low intensity training
   c. 7-12g/kg of BW should be ingested for optimal daily recovery from moderate to heavy endurance training
   d. 10-12g/kg of BW should be ingested for optimal daily recovery from an extreme exercise program

5. Which of the following is considered a reference for measuring the GI value of a specific food?

   a. White rice
   b. White bread
   c. Baked potato
   d. Enriched pasta

6. Which of the following is incorrectly listed as a disadvantage associated with using the classical supercompensation method to maximize glycogen stores in the days before competition?

    a.   Poor recovery when no CHO is ingested
    b.   Tenseness and anxiety from a week without regular training
    c.   Hyperglycemia can occur during the low-CHO period
    d.   Gastrointestinal problems during the high-protein, high-fat diet

7. Which of the following is the best recommendation related to carbohydrate intake hours before exercise or competition?

    a.   Ingest approximately 100g to 300g of CHO in a meal 5 to 6 hours before exercise or competition
    b.   Ingest approximately 140g to 330g of CHO in a meal 3 to 5 hours before exercise or competition
    c.   Ingest approximately 50g to 100g of CHO in a meal 2 to 3 hours before exercise or competition
    d.   Ingest approximately 140g to 330g of CHO in a meal 1 to 2 hours before exercise or competition

8. Which of the following would cause reactive hypoglycemia?

    a.   Ingestion of a high-protein, high-fat meal 3 hours prior to exercise
    b.   Ingestion of a very-high CHO meal directly after exercise
    c.   Ingestion of a moderate-sized, CHO-based meal 2 hours prior to exercise
    d.   Ingestion of a CHO-based meal 30 minutes prior to exercise

9. Which of the following is the optimal rate of CHO ingestion during prolonged exercise?

    a.   30g of CHO every hour (0.5g/min)
    b.   50g of CHO every hour (0.8g/min)
    c.   70g of CHO every hour (1.2g/min)
    d.   90g of CHO every hour (1.5g/min)

10. Which of the following statements concerning post-exercise CHO intake for maximal glycogen restoration is INCORRECT?

    a.   Post-exercise intake should occur as quickly as possible
    b.   The initial post-exercise meal should be a low-glycemic food
    c.   A small amount of protein in a post-exercise meal can improve recovery
    d.   The addition of caffeine may increase CHO delivery to muscle

SECTION 5 • <u>**CHECK YOUR WORK**</u>

SPORT NUTRITION CHAPTER 6 ANSWERS

<u>Match the Following Terms</u>

1. H	5. A	9. B
2. C	6. F	10. D
3. J	7. E	
4. I	8. G	

<u>Knowledge and Competency Exercises</u>

11. **Possible answers:** lactate, glycerol, pyruvate, amino acids

12. True

13. 1g or 4.0-4.5mmol

14. Hypoglycemia

15. **Possible answers:** a) consume 5-12g/kg depending on exercise intensity and duration, choose moderate to high-GI CHOs for the majority of immediate recovery meals (within 1-2 hours), b) consume a CHO-rich sports drink within the first hour after exercise when the appetite is suppressed, c) choose foods that also provide some protein during recovery meals to promote additional glycogen recovery, d) when training sessions are spaced less than 8 hours apart, begin CHO intake as quickly as possible; a series of snacks can help to meet demand, e) during longer recovery periods (24 hours) the athlete should organize the pattern and timing of CHO-rich foods according to what is practical and comfortable based on the situation, f) adequate total daily energy intake must be attained

16. Examples found on pages 129-130

17. 20%, ≥90 min

18. **Possible answers:** a) maintenance of blood glucose, b) greater CHO oxidation rates, c) glycogen sparing in the liver, d) promotion of glycogen synthesis, e) positive effects on motor skills, f) beneficial central nervous system effects

19. True

20. Possible answers: a) 1 L of a well-designed sports drinks (Gatorade, Powerade), b) 600 ml cola drink, c) 1.5 Power bars or Gatorade energy bars, d) 3 medium bananas, e) approximately 3 energy gels

Assess Your Knowledge

1. D

2. C

3. B

4. A

5. B

6. C

7. B

8. D

9. C

10. B

SECTION 1 • LEARNING GOALS

Upon completing this section, along with its corresponding chapter, you should understand the following:

1. The energy storage forms of fat in the human body

2. Sources of fatty acids (FAs) for use in the mitochondrion during exercise

3. The potential limiting factors during the process of fat oxidation

4. The factors which determine the rate of fat utilization during exercise

5. The relationship between CHO and fat utilization during exercise

6. The concepts related to fat supplementation before or during exercise

7. The effects of dieting plans such as fasting and high-fat diets on fat metabolism and performance

8. Supplemental claims related to enhanced FA utilization or mobilization

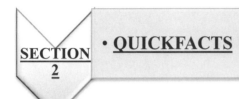

• QUICKFACTS

FAT STORAGE IN THE BODY

- Fat stores can provide 50x the amount of energy found in carbohydrate (CHO) stores (~100,000 Kcal)
- In theory, fat stores could provide energy for an average-sized runner to cover at least 1,300 km (~807 miles)
- Primary storage forms:
    - Plasma fatty acids (FA)
    - Plasma triacylglycerols (triglycerides)
    - Intramuscular triglycerides (IMTGs)
    - Adipose tissue – subcutaneous and visceral

Learn More: Sport Nutrition Textbook pg 150

FAT METABOLISM DURING EXERCISE

- FAs used during exercise are derived from several sources:
- **Triglycerides in adipose tissue** – split into FAs and glycerol
    - Glycerol is released into circulation and transported to the liver to produce glucose
    - FAs are either released into circulation and transported to working muscle or remain in adipose tissue to form new triglycerides (**reesterification)**
- **Circulating free FAs and triglycerides** such as very low-density lipoproteins (VLDL) can be pulled from circulation into working muscle
- **IMTGs** – split by hormone-sensitive lipase (HSL) to liberate FAs for transport into the mitochondrion

Learn More: Sport Nutrition Textbook pgs 150-151

POTENTIAL LIMITS TO FAT OXIDATION

- Fat utilization can be limited during any component of fat metabolism including:
    - **Lipolysis** – breakdown of triglycerides to FAs and glycerol
        - Dictated by enzyme and adrenal hormone action driven by the sympathetic nervous system (SNS) (e.g. catecholamines such as epinephrine, norepinephrine, dopamine)
        - At rest, 70% of the FAs are reesterified; during exercise this process is suppressed

- o **Removal of FAs from adipose tissue**
  - Dictated by blood flow to adipose tissue and concentration of the primary FA transporter **albumin** (99.9% of FA transport)
- o **Transport of fat by the bloodstream**
  - Serum triglycerides are metabolized by lipoprotein lipase secreted from the vascular wall for absorption in capillary beds
- o **Transport of FAs into the muscle cell**
  - Protein carriers function to transport FAs across the sarcolemma; muscle contractions increase carrier concentration
- o **Transport of FAs into the mitochondria**
  - IMTGs are usually located adjacent to mitochondria; can rapidly send liberated FAs for energy production
  - FAs in muscle cytoplasm are enzymatically triggered to form an acetyl-CoA complex (referred to as activated FAs) and bind to carnitine to enter the mitochondria
- o **Oxidation of the FAs in the β-oxidation pathway or tricarboxylic acid (TCA) cycle**
  - Dictated by enzymatic action and the presence of O_2

Learn More: Sport Nutrition Textbook pgs 151-155

FAT AS A FUEL DURING EXERCISE

- Multiple factors determine fat utilization during exercise:
  - o **Exercise intensity** – fat is the predominant fuel at lower intensities; maximal use is seen at 62%-63% of VO_2max; use increases as intensity increases (>65% VO_2max) but the percentage of contribution actually decreases

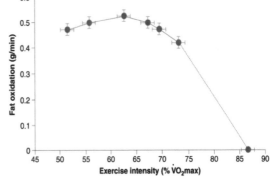

  - During exercise above 75% of VO_2max, use decreases to negligible levels as blood flow to adipose tissue is reduced and lactate accumulation increases the rate of reesterification
  - During very low-intensity exercise (25% of VO_2max), the majority of energy is derived from plasma FAs
  - During moderate intensity exercise (65% of VO_2max) IMTGs contribute to energy
  - o **Exercise duration** – fat oxidation increases with duration due to a decrease in glycogen
  - o **Diet** – a high-fat, low-CHO diet increases fat use; low-fat diet increases CHO use
  - o **CHO intake before exercise** – insulin action reduces lipolysis and FA use
  - o **Level of aerobic fitness** – fat oxidation is enhanced in aerobically trained individuals due to multiple adaptations:
    - Increased mitochondrial density and oxidative enzymes in trained muscle
    - Increased capillary density
    - Increased FA transporter concentrations in the sarcolemma of muscle

- Increased enzymatic action that promotes carnitine binding and FA transport into the mitochondria

Learn More: Sport Nutrition Textbook pgs 155-162

REGULATION OF CARBOHYDRATE AND FAT METABOLISM DURING EXERCISE

- Fat metabolism during exercise is regulated by CHO metabolism, but no specific mechanisms match FA use to energy expenditure; increased CHO use = reduced FA use and vice versa

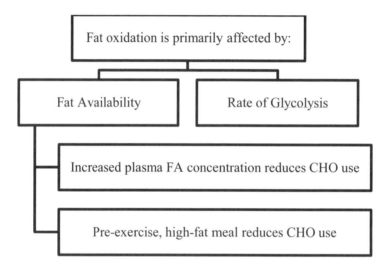

- CHO is the primary fuel for exercise, FAs appear to be more important during resting conditions

Learn More: Sport Nutrition Textbook pgs 159-162

FAT SUPPLEMENTATION BEFORE OR DURING EXERCISE

- Nutritional fats include long-chain triglycerides (LCTs), medium-chain triglycerides (MCTs), phospholipids, dietary cholesterol, and various oils
- Supplementation is aimed at sparing glycogen, but only LCTs and MCTs can contribute to energy during exercise
  - o Ingestion of LCTs during exercise is not desirable however:
    - They slow gastric emptying
    - They are absorbed and released into circulation at a very slow rate (3-4 hours)
    - They enter systemic circulation in chylomicrons, believed to be an insignificant fuel source during exercise
  - o MCTs are not commonly found in natural food sources but are marketed as a popular supplement among bodybuilders, they are not preferentially stored in the body but can provide significant energy
    - MCTs ingestion during exercise can be warranted as they are rapidly emptied from the stomach, absorbed, and oxidized; however, ingestion of large amounts can result in gastrointestinal distress

o   Fish oil has been shown to improve cellular membrane function and provide omega-3 essential FAs but does not appear to be an ergogenic fuel source

Learn More: Sport Nutrition Textbook pgs 162-163

EFFECT OF DIET ON FAT METABOLISM AND PERFORMANCE

- **Fasting** – increases availability of lipid substrates and FA oxidation at rest or during exercise, but as liver glycogen stores are not maintained, causes early fatigue and impaired performance during training $\geq$50% of VO$_2$max
    - o   Aerobic exercise employed after overnight fast enhances fat use (30 min steady state exercise)
- **Short-term, high-fat diet** – increases availability of lipid substrates and FA oxidation similar to fasting, but also reduces glycogen stores to an extent; higher intensity exercise performance is compromised
- **Long-term, high-fat diet** – chronic high-fat diets might increase the capacity to oxidize fat through enzymatic adaptations and spare glycogen use during exercise, but little evidence clearly indicates improved performance during competition

Learn More: Sport Nutrition Textbook pgs 163-66

SUPPLEMENTATION FOR INCREASED FAT OXIDATION

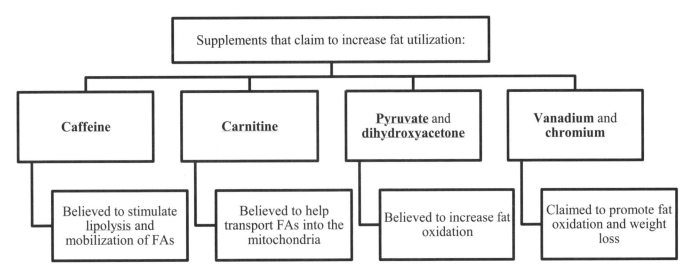

Learn More: Sport Nutrition Textbook pg 166

• <u>REVIEW YOUR KNOWLEDGE</u>

<u>Match the Following Terms</u>

1. _____ Reesterification   a. Liberates FAs from IMTGs within muscle tissue

2. _____ Intramuscular triglycerides   b. The breakdown of triglycerides into FAs and glycerol

3. _____ Hormone-sensitive lipase   c. Acetyl-CoA is split in the mitochondria to produce ATP

4. _____ Carnitine   d. Used in the liver to produce new glucose

5. _____ Lipolysis   e. Process where new triglycerides are formed in adipose tissue

6. _____ β-oxidation pathway   f. Typically located adjacent to mitochondria in muscle tissue

7. _____ Glycerol   g. Transport FAs into the mitochondria

<u>Knowledge and Competency Exercises</u>

8. List the four major storage forms of fat in the human body <u>in order</u> from lowest potential energy storage to greatest potential energy storage.

a) _____

b) _____

c) _____

d) _____

9. True or False? *(circle one)* During resting conditions, 30% of FAs are reesterified inside adipose tissue.

10. _____ muscle fibers have a greater concentration of IMTGs which are typically located adjacent to _____ within the tissue.

11. List four adaptations that promote enhanced fat oxidation in the muscle tissue of aerobically-trained individuals.

a) _____

b) _____

c) _____

d) _____

12. True or False? *(circle one)* CHO intake before exercise reduces FA utilization during exercise.

13. What two major factors regulate fat metabolism during exercise?

a) _____

b) _____

14. MCTs are popular among bodybuilders as they are not _____ and provide significant _____.

15. True or False? *(circle one)* Fish oil has been shown to improve cellular membrane function and provides omega-6 essential fatty acids.

• ASSESS YOUR KNOWLEDGE

SECTION 4

1. Triglycerides are broken down into which of the following to be used for energy?

    a. Enzymes and cholesterol
    b. Fatty acids and glycerol
    c. Glucose and polyunsaturated fatty acids
    d. Ketone bodies and ATP

2. Which of the following is not a source from which FAs can be derived and then utilized during exercise?

    a. Adipose tissue triglycerides
    b. Circulation
    c. IMTGs
    d. Glycerol

3. Which of the following is the primary transporter for FAs in the bloodstream?

    a. Carnitine
    b. Plasma triglycerides
    c. Very low-density lipoproteins (VLDLs)
    d. Albumin

4. Which of the following is <u>not</u> a step involved in fat metabolism?

    a. Adrenal hormones stimulate lipolysis in adipose tissue to liberate FAs and glycerol
    b. FAs are removed from adipose with adequate blood flow and albumin concentration
    c. Protein carriers function to transport FAs across the sarcolemma of muscle cells
    d. FAs in muscle cytoplasm are enzymatically triggered to form carnitine

5. Maximal fat utilization during exercise is seen at approximately what intensity?

    a. 40% of VO_2max
    b. 50% of VO_2max
    c. 60% of VO_2max
    d. 70% of VO_2max

6. Which of the following would <u>not</u> promote increased fat utilization as a fuel during exercise?

    a. Lower level of aerobic fitness
    b. Lower exercise intensity
    c. Longer exercise duration
    d. Engaging in a high-fat, low-CHO diet

7. Which of the following forms of nutritional fat can contribute to energy during exercise?

    a. Phospholipids
    b. Cholesterol
    c. MCTs
    d. Fish oil

8. Which of the following is an undesirable effect of LCT ingestion during exercise?

    a. They slow gastric emptying
    b. They are released into circulation at a very slow rate
    c. They enter circulation bound to chylomicrons which are believed to be an insignificant fuel source
    d. All of the above

9. Which of the following selections related to fasting is <u>incorrect</u>?

    a. Fasting increases the availability of lipid substrates
    b. Fasting significantly reduces performance at high intensities
    c. Fasting decreases FA oxidation at rest and during exercise
    d. Fasting lowers liver glycogen stores

10. Which of the following supplements is believed to stimulate lipolysis and enhance mobilization of FAs?

    a. Pyruvate
    b. Chromium
    c. Carnitine
    d. Caffeine

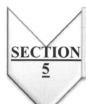

• **CHECK YOUR WORK**

SPORT NUTRITION CHAPTER 7 ANSWERS

Match the Following Terms

1. E	4. G	7. D
2. F	5. B	
3. A	6. C	

Knowledge and Competency Exercises

8. **a)** Plasma FAs, **b)** plasma triglycerides, **c)** intramuscular triglycerides (IMTGs), **d)** adipose tissue

9. False

10. Type I, mitochondria

11. **a)** Increased mitochondrial density and oxidative enzymes in trained muscle, **b)** increased capillary density, **c)** increased FA transporter concentrations in sarcolemma of muscle,

d) increased enzymatic action that promotes carnitine binding and FA transport into the mitochondria

12. True

13. **a)** Fat availability, **b)** the rate of CHO utilization

14. Preferentially stored in the body, energy

15. False

Assess Your Knowledge

1. B	5. C	9. C
2. D	6. A	10. D
3. D	7. C	
4. D	8. D	

- Protein turnover serves three main purposes:
    1. It degrades potentially damaged proteins to prevent a decline in their function
    2. Energy is provided when individual amino acids are converted into acetyl-CoA or TCA-cycle intermediates and oxidized in the mitochondria
    3. Individual amino acids can be used for the synthesis of other protein compounds such as neurotransmitters, hormones, creatine, and peptides, or other non-protein compounds such as fatty acids (FAs), glucose, ketones (which facilitate many reactions), or storage fat
- Before amino acids can be used in the TCA cycle to contribute to energy expenditure (EE), the amino group must be removed; this can occur in two ways:
    o **Transamination** – removal of the amino group by transferring it to a free **keto-acid**, which then forms a different amino acid
    o **Oxidative deamination** – amino group can be removed to form free ammonia (NH_3) which is either used to form glutamine within muscle or is transported to the liver to be converted into urea and excreted by the kidneys

Learn More: Sport Nutrition Textbook pgs 171-173, 175

TECHNIQUES TO STUDY PROTEIN AND AMINO ACID METABOLISM

- The following methods have been employed to study protein metabolism within the body to better understand protein intake needs:
    1. **Urea concentration in urine and sweat** – indicates whole-body protein breakdown
    2. **3-methylhistidine in urine and blood** – indicates contractile protein (myofibrillar) breakdown
    3. **Nitrogen balance** – widely used to determine recommended dietary intakes for protein; nitrogen intake is compared to nitrogen content in sweat, feces, and urine
        - When nitrogen intake exceeds nitrogen excretion the individual is in a positive nitrogen balance and must be retaining nitrogen and therefore protein
        - When nitrogen excretion exceeds nitrogen intake the individual is in a negative nitrogen balance and must be losing protein – this promotes muscle and organ catabolism to regain balance
    4. **Arteriovenous measurements of amino acids across a tissue bed** – can indicate nitrogen balance in a specific area of the body
    5. **Tracer methods** – labeled tracers are ingested or infused to follow specific amino acids in the body; have identical properties to the amino acid they trace but may emit radiation (radioactive isotopes) or are slightly heavier (stable isotopes)

Learn More: Sport Nutrition Textbook pgs 176-179

PROTEIN REQUIREMENTS FOR EXERCISE

| Protein requirements are believed to be greater for athletes because: |

| Amino acids may be oxidized during exercise | Increased protein synthesis is necessary to repair damage and forms the basis of training adaptations |

- It is estimated that protein contributes about 5%-15% to energy expenditure at rest; during exercise this drops to below 5% due to greater carbohydrate (CHO) and fat metabolism; only when available CHO is limited such as during starvation or prolonged exercise does protein use rise to around 10%
- **Recommended daily protein intake for endurance athletes** – 1.2-1.8g/kg of BW, in extreme cases it may rise to as high as 2.5g/kg of BW (Tour de France)
- **Recommended daily protein intake for strength athletes** – 1.6-1.7g/kg of BW, about twice the value for the general population – excess protein forms triglycerides

Learn More: Sport Nutrition Textbook pgs 179-180

PROTEIN INTAKE AMONG ATHLETES

- Most athletes consume ample protein to meet training needs as protein intake automatically increases with increased food intake
- Reported daily protein intake among athletes varies greatly - from below 0.8g/kg of BW among gymnasts to above 3.0g/kg of BW among bodybuilders

Learn More: Sport Nutrition Textbook pgs 180-182

PROTEIN INTAKE AND SYNTHESIS

- After exercise, protein synthesis and breakdown increase; synthesis will only surpass breakdown when amino acids are ingested
- If feeding is delayed for several hours net protein balance remains negative and muscle hypertrophy is inhibited
- Key factors that affect protein synthesis after exercise:
    1. **Coingestion of other nutrients** – CHO ingestion with the protein increases plasma insulin concentrations which may cause a reduction in protein breakdown
    2. **The amount of protein** – research suggests around 20g-25g is required

Athletes at increased risk for protein deficiency: Female runners, Male wrestlers, Athletes in weight category sports, Ski jumpers, Male and female gymnasts, Female dancers, Vegetarians

3. **The timing of protein intake** – CHO and amino acids ingested immediately prior to exercise seems to promote the greatest protein synthesis and amino acid uptake (6g of essential amino acids, 35g of carbohydrate used in one study),while controlled amounts of whey protein ingested alone provides the same effect when ingested either before or 1-3 hours after exercise

4. **The type of protein** – fast-absorbing proteins (essential amino acids as opposed to whey) seem to be optimal for synthesis; certain types have been shown to be superior compared to others in certain situations (e.g., effect of milk vs. soy and muscle mass gains in bodybuilders) but more research is needed to discern the best type in each training scenario

Learn More: Sport Nutrition Textbook pgs 182-184

AMINO ACIDS AS ERGOGENIC AIDS

The following amino acids are marketed to assist in various components of sports performance:

- **Arginine** – functions to facilitate anabolic effects
  - *Claims* – improves immune function, increases creatine levels, increases release of insulin and growth hormone, lead to fewer gastrointestinal problems
  - *Proven effects* – large dosage injections increase the release of growth hormone, but oral dosages cannot be tolerated at the quantity necessary for this reaction; other claims have limited supporting evidence
- **Aspartate** – precursor for TCA-cycle intermediates that reduces fatigue-causing plasma ammonia accumulation during exercise
  - *Claims* – improves energy metabolism in muscle, reduces amount of fatigue-causing metabolites, improves endurance performance
  - *Proven effects* – supplementation has not been shown to increase exercise time to exhaustion
- **BCAAs** – includes the essential amino acids leucine, isoleucine, and valine; oxidized during exercise
  - *Claims* – provide fuel for working muscle, reduce fatigue, improve endurance, reduce muscle protein breakdown
  - *Proven effects* – all claims have limited supporting evidence as many foods provide significant quantities of BCAAs; consuming BCAAs over daily need does not improve performance when adequate protein is consumed, but BCAA and the other essential amino acids may aid in protein uptake when consumed with appropriate quantities of CHO immediately prior to exercise
    - (e.g., one chicken breast (100g) provides the equivalent of about seven BCAA doses)
- **Glutamine** – functions as a constituent of proteins, a means of nitrogen transport between tissues, an antioxidant precursor, and facilitates other immunological and metabolic reactions
  - *Claims* – improves immune function, promotes rapid water absorption from the gut, hastens recovery after exercise, improves performance, leads to fewer gastrointestinal problems
  - *Proven effects* – limited evidence demonstrates slightly improved glycogen synthesis after exercise; other claims have no supporting evidence
- **Glycine** – involved in the synthesis of phosphocreatine
  - *Claims* – increases phosphocreatine synthesis, improves sprint performance, increases strength
  - *Proven effects* – claims remain unconfirmed
- **Ornithine** – suggested to stimulate growth hormone from the pituitary gland

- *Claims* – increases growth hormone and insulin release, stimulates protein synthesis, reduces protein breakdown, improves performance
- *Proven effects* – injection stimulates an even greater release of growth hormone than arginine but supplement forms do not appear to be effective

- **Taurine** – non-protein AA, concentrations are high in the brain and heart but role is poorly understood; theorized to act as a membrane stabilizer, an antioxidant, and a neuromodulator – common ingredient (1000 mg) in energy drinks
  - *Claims* – delays fatigue, improves performance, facilitates faster recovery, leads to less muscle damage and pain, leads to fewer gastrointestinal problems, scavenges free radicals
  - *Proven effects* – claims remain unconfirmed and synergistic effects unclear

- **Tryptophan** – precursor of the neurotransmitter serotonin
  - *Claims* – increases the release of growth hormone, improves sleep, decreases sensations of pain, improves performance
  - *Proven effects* – claims related to exercise lack significant evidence, elevated doses may negatively affect prolonged exercise performance

- **Tyrosine** – ingestion increases circulating concentrations of epinephrine, norepinephrine, and dopamine
  - *Claims* – increases blood concentration of catecholamines which improves fuel mobilization and metabolism during exercise
  - *Proven effects* – large dosages not commonly seen in marketed supplements (5g-10g vs. 100mg) have been shown to prevent the substantial decline in various aspects of cognitive performance and mood associated with acute stress such as choice reaction time and pattern recognition; controlled studies have failed to demonstrate positive effects on exercise performance

Learn More: Sport Nutrition Textbook pgs 184-191

PROTEIN INTAKE AND HEALTH RISKS

- Excessive intake of more than 3g/kg of BW has been claimed to have various negative physiological effects such as:
  - Kidney damage
  - Increased cholesterol and risk for atherosclerosis
  - Dehydration
- Dehydration – increased nitrogen excretion in urine results in increased urinary volume and fluid loss, therefore additional fluid intake is warranted with increased protein intake
- In healthy people with no indication of kidney issues there is no clear evidence that high protein intake near the UL is dangerous, but fluid intake should be increased
- For most athletes, the biggest danger of high protein intake is that it often comes at the cost of CHO intake

Learn More: Sport Nutrition Textbook pg 191

SECTION 3   • REVIEW YOUR KNOWLEDGE

Match the Following Terms

1. _____ Nonessential amino acids   a. Reduces plasma ammonia accumulation during exercise

2. _____ Arginine   b. Promotes growth hormone release

3. _____ Tyrosine   c. Process of bodily protein breakdown into free amino acids

4. _____ Protein synthesis   d. Transfer of an amino group to a free keto-acid

5. _____ Aspartate   e. Increases circulating epinephrine

6. _____ Protein degradation   f. Involved in the synthesis of phosphocreatine

7. _____ Glycine   g. Are synthesized within the human body

8. _____ Transamination   h. Concentrations are very high in the brain and heart

9. _____ Taurine   i. Process of free amino acid assimilation into bodily proteins

10. _____ Tryptophan   j. May improve sleep as a precursor of serotonin

Knowledge and Competency Exercises

11. List four forms of amino acids and proteins found in the human body.

a) _____

b) _____

c) _____

d) _____

12. Free amino acid carriers recognize an amino acid's specific _____ and _____to allow for their transport into tissues.

13. True or False? (*circle one*) Individual amino acids can be used for the synthesis of neurotransmitters, hormones, creatine, fatty acids, glucose, or ketones.

14. Fill in the missing data in the following table related to methods for estimating protein metabolism.

Method	Advantages	Disadvantages and Limitations
Nitrogen balance	Accurate when used over relatively long periods	
	No health risk	Relatively expensive; sophisticated equipment needed
Arteriovenous measurements of amino acids across a tissue bed		Invasive; has high variability, depends on blood flow
Urea concentration in urine and sweat		

15. True or False? (*circle one*) When nitrogen intake exceeds nitrogen excretion the individual is in a positive nitrogen balance and must be retaining protein.

16. List two reasons why protein requirements are believed to be greater for athletes.

a) _____

b) _____

17. Identify three athletic populations that may be at increased risk for protein deficiency.

a) _____

b) _____

c) _____

18. True or False? (*circle one*) In the hours following exercise, protein synthesis will surpass protein breakdown only when amino acids are ingested.

19. True or False? (*circle one*) Supplementing BCAAs has not been proven to enhance exercise performance beyond consuming the same quantity of essential amino acids in natural food products.

20. Supplemental _____ is marketed to improve immune function, promote rapid water absorption from the gut, hasten recovery after exercise, and lead to fewer gastrointestinal problems; but none of these claims have been clearly demonstrated in research.

SECTION 4 • **ASSESS YOUR KNOWLEDGE**

1. Which of the following is the most abundant free amino acid in muscle and blood plasma?

    a. BCAA
    b. Arginine
    c. Glutamine
    d. Taurine

2. Which of the following is not a function of protein turnover within the human body?

    a. The degradation of damaged proteins prevents a decline in their function
    b. Energy provision
    c. Synthesis of necessary compounds such as neurotransmitters and hormones
    d. Stimulate the liberation of glycerol from adipose and intramuscular triglycerides

3. When an amino acid undergoes oxidative deamination to enter the TCA cycle for energy, which of the following compounds is formed as a byproduct that must be excreted by the kidneys?

    a. Epinephrine
    b. Ammonia (NH_3)
    c. Keto-acids
    d. Ketones

4. Which of the following describes what will occur when an individual remains in a negative nitrogen balance?

    a. Muscle fiber hypertrophy
    b. Kidney damage
    c. Liver damage
    d. Muscle and organ atrophy

5. To what degree can protein contribute to energy expenditure in extreme cases of prolonged exercise?

    a. Up to 10% of energy expenditure
    b. Up to 20% of energy expenditure
    c. Up to 30% of energy expenditure
    d. Up to 40% of energy expenditure

6. What is the recommended daily intake of protein for strength athletes?

    a. 1.2-1.5g/kg of BW
    b. 1.4-1.6g/kg of BW
    c. 1.6-1.7g/kg of BW
    d. 1.8-2.0g/kg of BW

7. Which of the following would not have an optimal effect on protein synthesis occurring after an intense bout of resistance training?

    a. Ingestion of CHO with protein intake directly after the exercise bout
    b. Ingestion of 25g of essential amino acids five hours after the exercise bout
    c. Ingestion of 6g of essential amino acids with 35g of CHO immediately prior to the exercise bout
    d. Ingestion of 20g of essential amino acids one hour after the exercise bout

8. Which of the following amino acids marketed as a supplement has been shown, when administered in large doses, to prevent the substantial decline in various aspects of cognitive performance and mood when encountering acute stress?

    a. Tyrosine
    b. Taurine
    c. Ornithine
    d. Tryptophan

9. Which of the following amino acids is known to help synthesize antioxidants and facilitate immunological functions?

    a. Arginine
    b. Aspartate
    c. Glutamine
    d. Glycine

10. Which of the following statements related to protein intake and health risks is incorrect?

    a. For many athletes the biggest danger of high protein intake is that it often comes at the cost of reduced CHO intake
    b. Increased protein intake may promote direct negative effects on blood cholesterol
    c. Athletes on a high protein diet need to consume more fluids due to the increased demand to flush out excess nitrogen in the urine
    d. Healthy people with no indications of kidney issues can consume higher protein intakes

SPORT NUTRITION CHAPTER 8 ANSWERS

<u>Match the Following Terms</u>

1. G	5. A	9. H
2. B	6. C	10. J
3. E	7. F	
4. I	8. D	

<u>Knowledge and Competency Exercises</u>

11. **a)** pool of free amino acids in circulation, **b)** blood protein structures, **c)** viscera, **d)** skeletal muscle and connective tissues

12. **a)** shape, **b)** chemical properties

13. True

14.

Method	Advantages	Disadvantages and Limitations
Nitrogen balance	Accurate when used over relatively long periods	**Difficult and time consuming; tends to overestimate nitrogen retention, usually ignores loss in sweat**
Stable isotopes	No health risk	Relatively expensive; sophisticated equipment needed
Arteriovenous measurements of amino acids across a tissue bed	**Gives data on net exchange of amino acids, net uptake of essential amino acids related to rate of protein synthesis**	Invasive; has high variability, depends on blood flow
Urea concentration in urine and sweat	**Easy, relatively cheap**	**Only rough estimate; heavily affected by diet**

15. True

16. **a)** amino acids may be oxidized during exercise, **b)** increased protein synthesis is necessary to repair damage and forms the basis of training adaptations

17. **Possible answers**: female runners, male wrestlers, boxers and other athletes in weight category sports, ski jumpers, male and female gymnasts, female dancers, vegetarians

18. True

19. True

20. Glutamine

Assess Your Knowledge

1. C

2. D

3. B

4. D

5. A

6. C

7. B

8. A

9. C

10. B

SECTION 1   • **LEARNING GOALS**

Upon completing this section, along with its corresponding chapter, you should understand the following:

1. Concepts and definitions related to hydration

2. Concepts related to daily water balance within the body

3. The effects of exercise on body temperature

4. The modes by which the body can gain or lose heat while encountering environmental heat stress

5. Concepts related to thermoregulation and water loss during exercise

6. The optimal method for assessing environmental heat stress

7. The physiological mechanisms that allow for temperature regulation during exercise

8. The means by which the body acclimates to training in the heat

9. The effects of dehydration on exercise performance

10. The physiological mechanisms and major risk factors behind heat injury

11. The benefits of optimal hydration and hyperhydration on exercise performance

12. The challenges athletes face in attaining optimal fluid consumption during exercise

13. The fluid intake recommendations for athletes to follow for optimal hydration prior to, during, and after prolonged exercise or athletic competition

• QUICKFACTS

WATER AND HYDRATION

- Sufficient water intake is required to maintain health and physical performance; no intake for only a few days results in death
- **Hydration** – relates to the balance between water intake and water loss
- **Dehydration** – reduction in body's water content, significantly impairs physical performance
- **Euhydration** – normal state of total body water
- **Hypohydration** – reduction in total body water
- **Hyperhydration** – intake of extra water; when properly employed, enhances blood volume and can limit the decline in performance in hot environments
- Water accounts for 50%-60% of body mass; lean mass dictates total content
    o Lean body tissues contain about 75% by mass
    o Adipose contains about 5% by mass

Learn More: Sport Nutrition Textbook pg 196

DAILY WATER BALANCE

- Water loss occurs through:
    ➢ Respiration
    ➢ Skin – evaporation of sweat
    ➢ Feces
    ➢ Urine
- Water gain occurs through:
    ➢ Ingestion of fluids
    ➢ Ingestion of food
    ➢ Metabolic breakdown of macronutrients
- Environmental factors and daily activity level dictate water loss, and consequently, the necessary fluid intake to maintain balance

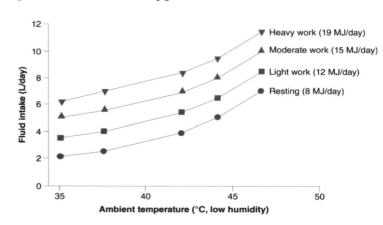

Learn More: Sport Nutrition Textbook pgs 211-213

EXERCISE AND BODY TEMPERATURE

- A body temperature of 36-38 °C (96.8-100.4 °F) is considered normal during rest
- Temperature may increase to 38-40 °C (100.4-104 °F) during exercise
- Central fatigue occurs when temperature reaches 39.5 °C (103 °F); further increases are commonly associated with heat illness
- **Thermoregulation** – important internal mechanisms that prevent **hyperthermia**, or a potentially dangerous rise in body temperature
    - Example: Training at 80%-90% of VO_2max could increase body temperature by 1 °C every 4-5 minutes if no changes occurred in the body's heat dissipating mechanisms
- **Heat production during exercise** – muscular work produces excess heat that is transferred to the core to keep working musculature cool enough to continue contracting
    - The greater the O_2 use (intensity), the greater the increase in heat production
- **Heat storage during exercise** – elevated core temperature is caused by a temporary imbalance between the rates of heat production and dissipation during the early stages of exercise

Learn More: Sport Nutrition Textbook pgs 197-198

ENVIRONMENTAL HEAT STRESS

- Environmental heat stress is dictated by:
    - Ambient temperature
    - Relative humidity
    - Wind velocity
    - Solar radiation
- Modes by which heat is gained or lost during exercise:
- **Radiation** – transfer of heat by emission from one object and absorbed by another
    - *Example* – ground/sun can radiate heat which is absorbed by the body
- **Conduction** – transfer of heat from one object or substance into another to maintain a balanced temperature gradient
    - *Example* – body could transfer heat into a relatively cool bench used for rest
- **Convection** – exchange of heat between a solid object and one that moves
    - *Example* – body could transfer heat into relatively cool wind it contacts during movement
- **Evaporation** – the vaporization of a liquid; most important method of heat loss
    - *Example* – evaporation of sweat on the skin allows the dissipation of stored heat within the body into surrounding air

Learn More: Sport Nutrition Textbook pg 198-199

DYNAMICS OF THERMOREGULATION AND WATER LOSS DURING EXERCISE

- **Skin is hotter than its surroundings** – heat is dissipated into the environment by evaporation through sweating, convection, radiation, and conduction
- **Surroundings are hotter than the skin** – heat is absorbed by the body via convection and conduction
- **Surroundings are saturated with water vapor (humidity)** – evaporation of sweat is thwarted, resulting in reduced loss of heat
- Heavy sweating occurs during intense exercise to limit a rise in body temperature which leads to progressive dehydration and loss of electrolytes
- <u>Summary Concept:</u> High **ambient temperature** (loss of convection/conduction) and **high humidity** (loss of evaporation) = increased risk for **dehydration** and **hyperthermia**

Learn More: Sport Nutrition Textbook pg 198-199, 201

ASSESSING ENVIRONMENTAL HEAT STRESS

- A useful index of environmental heat stress is the **wet bulb globe temperature** (WBGT)

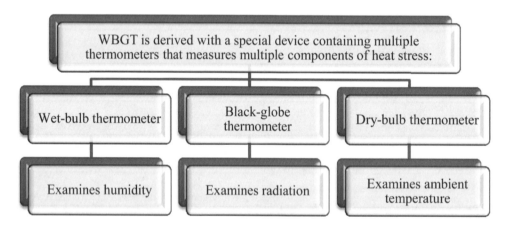

- Provides a comprehensive assessment of overall risk for heat injury in a given environment

Learn More: Sport Nutrition Textbook pg 198

PHYSIOLOGICAL REGULATION OF BODY TEMPERATURE

- Central control systems in the body receive data on heat stress in multiple ways:
  - Sensory data from thermoreceptors in the skin and core
  - Central thermoreceptors located in the hypothalamus can sense minute temperature changes within circulation to the brain
  - Nervous signals from osmoreceptors and pressure receptors can sense changes in plasma osmolarity and blood volume
- The hypothalamus is considered the "thermostat" of the body which can interpret sensory data and consequently stimulate the following reactions when encountering heat stress:
  1. **Cutaneous dilation** – to increase possible heat loss via radiation and convection

2. **Initiation of sweating** – to allow for evaporative heat loss
- Hormones and neurotransmitters such as estrogen, cytokines, dopamine, and noradrenaline are also capable of influencing thermoregulatory responses

Learn More: Sport Nutrition Textbook pg 200

EXERCISE, ACCLIMATIZATION, AND TEMPERATURE REGULATION

- Heat acclimation is attained by training at high intensities (70%-100% of VO_2max) in a hot environment
- Acclimation is not achieved by training at lower intensities or resting in a hot environment
- Repeated, intense training in the heat can improve thermoregulatory capabilities through the following adaptations:
    1. **An increase in blood volume**
    2. **An increase in the capacity for blood flow to the skin**
    3. **An increase in the size of sweat glands**
    4. **An earlier onset of sweating** (lower set-point core temperature)
    5. **An increase in sweat rate** (increased sensitivity of the relationship between sweat rate and core temperature)

Learn More: Sport Nutrition Textbook pgs 200-202

EFFECTS OF DEHYDRATION ON EXERCISE PERFORMANCE

- During prolonged training, dehydration may cause just as much fatigue as fuel depletion; its negative effects are more pronounced in hot environments
- Exercise performance is impaired by dehydration as low as 2% of BW; water loss in excess of 5% of BW can decrease the capacity for work by about 30%
    - Effect of dehydration on strength and power activities (lasting >30 sec but <2 min) is poorly understood but believed to reduce performance by 2%-3%
    - Clinical dehydration (2.5% of BW) can significantly reduce high-intensity interval sprinting performance, 45% reduction shown in research
    - Significant dehydration (7% of BW) has been shown to reduce total time to exhaustion even during walking
- Physiological effects that occur during dehydration which have an adverse effect on exercise performance:
    1. **Reduction in blood volume (hypovolemia)** – plasma lost in sweat
    2. **Decreased skin blood flow** – due to hypovolemia and subsequent reduction in cardiac output
    3. **Decreased heat dissipation** – impaired ability to sweat

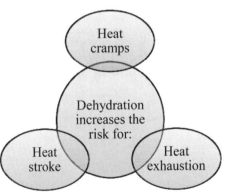

4. **Increased core temperature** – increased cardiovascular strain
5. **Increased rate of muscle glycogen use** – caused by release of increased stress hormones

Learn More: Sport Nutrition Textbook pgs 202-204

MECHANISMS OF HEAT INJURY

- Exhaustive training in a hot, humid environment (especially while dehydrated) can cause the following cascade of events leading to life-threatening heat injury:
1. Sweating begins and skin blood vessels dilate to increase heat loss
2. Pooling of blood in the periphery reduces central blood volume
3. Cardiac output is reduced from hypovolemia, increasing heart rate and cardiovascular strain
4. As central blood volume continues to drop, sympathetic nervous system activity causes vasoconstriction of skin and abdominal organ blood vessels
5. Lack of circulation to the skin impairs heat loss and core temperature rises
6. Lack of circulation to the gastrointestinal tract, liver, and kidneys results in cellular hypoxia and the production of **reactive oxygen species** (ROS)
7. ROS cause damage to cellular membranes, making them leaky; this can allow the passage of **endotoxins** (bacterial toxins) from the gastrointestinal tract into circulation
8. Circulating endotoxins lead to **endotoxemia** (blood poisoning) and a drastic fall in blood pressure
9. When core temperature reaches a critical level in conjunction with the previous issues, **heat syncope** (fainting) and organ injury can result

Learn More: Sport Nutrition Textbook pg 204-205

RISK OF HEAT ILLNESS

- Heat-related pathology contributes to poor health and mortality in athletes, elderly, children, and disabled populations; third-leading cause of death among U.S. high school athletes
- Significant risk factors for heat illness:
  - Dehydration – most common factor
  - Hot and humid climate
  - Obesity
  - Low physical fitness
  - Lack of acclimatization
  - Previous history of heat stroke
  - Sleep deprivation
  - Medications (particularly diuretics or antidepressants)
  - Sweat gland dysfunction
  - Upper respiratory or gastrointestinal illness

Learn More: Sport Nutrition Textbook pg 205

FLUID INTAKE AND EXERCISE PERFORMANCE

- Fluid intake during exercise helps restore plasma volume lost in sweat and prevent the adverse effects of dehydration on performance
- **Pre-exercise hyperhydration** – improves thermoregulation by expanding blood volume and reducing blood osmolarity; allows for improved heat dissipation
  - ➢ Studies have demonstrated increased sweating rates, lower core temperatures, and lower heart rates with proper implementation
  - ➢ Greater fluid retention during hyperhydration seems to be achieved if glycerol is added to pre-exercise fluids
- Ideally, athletes should consume enough fluids so that body weight remains constant before and after exercise

Learn More: Sport Nutrition Textbook pgs 205-206

FLUID INTAKE CHALLENGES

- **Fluid consumption must match sweat loss to avoid dehydration during exercise** but achieving this goal is difficult for a number of reasons:
  - o Sweat rates during strenuous exercise in the heat can reach 2-3 L/h, but more than about 1 L of fluid in the stomach is uncomfortable for most athletes; gastric emptying rate may not allow for a consumption/loss match to occur
  - o Sweat rates vary widely among individuals in the same ambient temperature, so prescribing an exact quantity of fluid to consume is difficult if the athlete has not trained in the specific environment before
  - o Relying on thirst as the signal to drink is not optimal as a degree of dehydration sufficient to impair athletic performance can occur before the desire for fluid intake is evident
  - o The rules or practicalities of a sport may limit the opportunities for drinking during competition

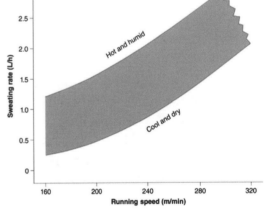

Learn More: Sport Nutrition Textbook pgs 207-208

OPTIMAL FLUID FOR PROLONGED EXERCISE

- Optimal characteristics of fluids consumed during prolonged events (>1hr):
  - ➢ Should be cooler than ambient temperature, flavored to enhance palatability, and non-carbonated
  - ➢ Should be ingested at a rate of 600-1,200 ml/hr in a solution containing 4%-8% CHO in the form of sugars (glucose or sucrose) or starch (maltodextrins) to provide energy while allowing for rapid gastric emptying and absorption

➢ Should not be hypertonic with respect to blood plasma as this will delay restoration of plasma volume (e.g., high CHO concentrations such as 16%)
➢ Should include sodium (500-700 mg/L of fluid) to increase palatability, promote fluid retention, and prevent hyponatremia (low serum sodium) with ingestion of large quantities of fluid

Learn More: Sport Nutrition Textbook pgs 208

FLUID INTAKE AND HYDRATION RECOMMENDATIONS FOR ATHLETES

- Recommendations for optimizing hydration levels prior to exercise or athletic competition:
  o Consume a balanced diet and drink adequate fluids during the 24 hours **prior to** the event
  o Inspect the color of the urine (which should be pale yellow) to help ensure proper hydration is maintained
  o Fluid intake of 6-8 ml/kg of BW about 2 hours before exercise should provide enough time for optimal fluid absorption and excretion of excess water
    ▪ Fluid with some sodium or salty snacks may stimulate thirst and help retain fluids
  o Alternate recommendation - drink 500 ml of fluid 2 hours before exertion and another 500 ml 15 minutes before the event
- Recommendations for optimizing hydration levels **during** exercise or athletic competition:
  o Begin drinking early and at regular intervals
  o Due to varying sweat rates amongst individuals, customized fluid replacement programs should be employed
  o Measurement of pre-exercise and post-exercise body weight is useful for determining sweat rates and developing a personal fluid intake program
- Recommendations for optimizing hydration levels **after** exercise or athletic competition:
  o For rapid and complete recovery from excessive dehydration, 1.5 L of fluid should be consumed for each kg of BW lost (essentially 150% of weight loss) to potentially achieve normal hydration within 6 hours
    ▪ The addition of sodium can aid recovery by stimulating thirst and fluid retention
  o Intake of caffeine and alcohol in the post-exercise recovery period is discouraged due to their diuretic actions

Learn More: Sport Nutrition Textbook pgs 208-217

SECTION 3 • REVIEW YOUR KNOWLEDGE

Match the Following Terms

1. _____ Dehydration		a. Loss of consciousness related to heat injury
2. _____ Wet bulb globe temperature		b. Exchange of heat between a solid object and one that moves
3. _____ Radiation		c. Can cause damage to cellular membranes making them leaky
4. _____ Hypothalamus		d. Potentially dangerous rise in body temperature
5. _____ Euhydration		e. Bacterial toxins from gut that can be released into circulation
6. _____ Reactive oxygen species		f. Transfer of heat by emission from one object to another
7. _____ Endotoxins		g. Reduction in body water content
8. _____ Convection		h. Comprehensive index of environmental heat stress
9. _____ Hyperthermia		i. The central thermal controller or "thermostat" of the body
10. _____ Heat syncope		j. Normal state of body water

Knowledge and Competency Exercises

11. True or False? (*circle one*) Water accounts for 50%-60% of total body mass with adipose tissue containing more water by mass than lean body tissues.

12. Fill in the following table concerning the modes by which body water is gained or lost on a daily basis.

WATER LOSS	WATER GAIN
1.	1.
2.	2.
3.	3.
4.	

13. _____ generally begins when body temperature reaches 39.5 °C (103 °F).

14. List four factors that directly dictate environmental heat stress.

a) _____   b) _____

c) _____   d) _____

15. True or False? (*circle one*) Body heat transferred into a relatively cool bench used to rest on during interval sprints is an example of conduction.

16. High ambient temperature and high humidity = high risk for _____ and _____ .

17. A wet bulb globe temperature (WBGT) is derived from a special device containing multiple thermometers that measures what specific components of heat stress?

a) _____   b) _____   c) _____

18. The hypothalamus, or thermostat of the body, can stimulate _____ and the initiation of _____ to allow for optimal dissipation of heat.

19. List five physiological effects that occur during dehydration which have an adverse effect on exercise performance.

a) _____

b) _____

c) _____

d) _____

e) _____

20. True or False? (*circle one*) Reliance on thirst as the signal to drink is not optimal as a degree of dehydration sufficient to impair performance can occur before the desire for fluid intake is evident.

• PRACTICAL APPLICATIONS

SECTION 4

1. An 80kg athlete participates in a 3-hour endurance event. He loses 3 kg during the event and feels like he did not perform at maximum capacity as he perceives he became dehydrated early on in the race. He also did not recover well and senses he should have employed a different nutritional strategy after the race.

(A) What recommendation(s) could have been provided to him related to fluid ingestion prior to the event to optimize hyperhydration?

_____

_____

_____

(B) What recommendation(s) could have been provided to him related to fluid ingestion during the event to thwart the progression of dehydration and fuel depletion?

_____

_____

_____

(C) What recommendation(s) could have been provided to him related to fluid intake after the event to optimize recovery?

_____

_____

_____

1. Environmental heat stress is dictated by each of the following except?

   a. Ambient temperature
   b. Core radiation
   c. Relative humidity
   d. Wind velocity

2. Which of the following modes of potential heat loss is severely limited when training in a humid environment?

   a. Radiation
   b. Conduction
   c. Convection
   d. Evaporation

3. How much water can a fit athlete potentially lose each hour in the form of sweat when engaging in strenuous training in a hot environment?

   a. 0.5 L/h
   b. 1.0 L/h
   c. 1.5-2.0 L/h
   d. 2.0-3.0 L/h

4. Which of the following is not a physiological adaptation that occurs as an athlete acclimates to training in the heat?

   a. Blood volume increases
   b. An earlier onset of sweating
   c. An increase in the number of sweat glands
   d. An increase in the capacity for blood flow to the skin

5. Water loss of 5% of total body weight can decrease the capacity for work by what percentage?

   a. 10%
   b. 20%
   c. 30%
   d. 40%

6. Which of the following issues is related to heat syncope?

   a. Endotoxemia
   b. Enhanced heat dissipation
   c. Hyperhydration
   d. Low electrolytes

7. Which of the following is <u>not</u> considered a risk factor for heat injury/illness?

   a. Obesity
   b. Excessive sleep (>10hrs)
   c. Low physical fitness
   d. Lack of acclimatization

8. Which of the following supplements may enhance fluid retention during hyperhydration?

   a. Caffeine
   b. Glutamine
   c. Glycerol
   d. Lactose

9. Which of the following is <u>not</u> an optimal attribute of fluid consumption during prolonged events (>1hour)?

   a. The fluid should be cooler than the ambient temperature
   b. Fluids should be ingested at a rate of 600-1,200 ml/h
   c. The fluid should contain sodium
   d. The fluid should be hypertonic with respect to blood plasma

10. Which of the following describes the optimal intake of fluids to allow for hyperhydration prior to a prolonged competitive event in the heat?

   a. The athlete should consume 1-2 ml of fluid per kilogram of BW about 2 hours prior to the event
   b. The athlete should consume 3-5 ml of fluid per kilogram of BW about 1 hour prior to the event
   c. The athlete should consume 6-8 ml of fluid per kilogram of BW about 2 hours prior to the event
   d. The athlete should consume 8-10 ml of fluid per kilogram of BW about 3 hours prior to the event

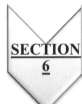

SECTION 6 • CHECK YOUR WORK

SPORT NUTRITION CHAPTER 9 ANSWERS

Match the Following Terms

1. G	5. J	9. D
2. H	6. C	10. A
3. F	7. E	
4. I	8. B	

Knowledge and Competency Exercises

11. False

12.

WATER LOSS	WATER GAIN
1. Respiration	1. Ingestion of fluids
2. Skin	2. Ingestion of food
3. Feces	3. Metabolic breakdown of macronutrients
4. Urine	

13. Central (brain) fatigue

14. **a)** Ambient temperature, **b)** relative humidity, **c)** wind velocity, **d)** solar radiation

15. True

16. Dehydration, hyperthermia

17. **a)** humidity, **b)** radiation, **c)** ambient temperature

18. Cutaneous dilation, sweating

19. **a)** Reduction in blood volume, **b)** decreased skin blood flow, **c)** decreased heat dissipation, **d)** increased core temperature, **e)** increased rate of muscle glycogen use

20. True

Practical Applications

1. (A) He should ingest about 6-8 ml of fluid per kilogram of BW about 2 hours before exercise to allow for optimal fluid absorption and excretion of excess water. Based on his body size, this would equate to approximately 480-640ml. The fluid should also contain some sodium to potentially enhance retention.

(B) He should ingest 600-1,200 ml/h in a solution containing 4%-8% CHO in the form of sugars (glucose or sucrose) or starch (maltodextrins) to provide energy while allowing for rapid gastric emptying and absorption. For this 3-hour event, his total fluid intake during the event would equate to approximately 1,800-3,600 ml.

(C) To promote rapid and complete recovery from excessive dehydration after exercise, 1.5 L of fluid should be consumed for each kilogram of BW lost (150% of weight loss); the addition of sodium will aid in recovery by stimulating thirst and fluid retention. Based on his weight loss during the event, he should have ingested 4.5 L of fluid in the first hour or so after the event.

Assess Your Knowledge

1. B	6. A
2. D	7. B
3. D	8. C
4. C	9. D
5. C	10. C

SECTION 1 • LEARNING GOALS

Upon completing this section, along with its corresponding chapter, you should understand the following:

1. The major functions of key water-soluble and fat-soluble vitamins as well as macrominerals and microminerals as they relate to physical performance

2. The risk factors for inadequate vitamin and mineral intake among athletes as well as specific groups at greater risk for dietary intake which negatively affects performance

3. Key micronutrients to consider during periods of elevated training due to elevated need and/or loss as a consequece of physical activity

4. The roles of micronutrients during tissue synthesis, immune function, electrolyte dynamics, and other enzymatic actions related to maintaining physiological homeostasis and performance

5. Issues related to mineral deficiency such as osteoporosis and anemia

6. The sources, functions, and protective mechanisms of antioxidants as well as the positive and negative effects of free radicals

7. The potential dangers of high-dose micronutrient supplementation

8. The methods employed and issues related to assessing micronutrient status among athletes

9. Micronutrient intake considerations for athletes related to attaining adequate calcium and iron, special issues such as amenorrhea, and training in hot and humid environments

• QUICKFACTS

FUNCTIONS OF VITAMINS AND MINERALS

- Vitamins and minerals do not directly contribute to energy supply but are necessary for the following processes:
    - Growth and repair of body tissues
    - Act as cofactors in metabolic energy-producing reactions
    - Oxygen transport and oxidative metabolism
    - Immune function
    - Act as antioxidants
- Any sustained deficiency of an essential vitamin or mineral will cause negative health effects; a deficient athlete is unlikely to be able to perform at maximum capacity

Learn More: Sport Nutrition Textbook pgs 222-224

WATER-SOLUBLE AND FAT-SOLUBLE VITAMINS

- There are 13 different vitamins including 4 fat-soluble and 9 water-soluble compounds
- Vitamin D, vitamin K, and small quantities of select B vitamins can be produced within the body; the rest can only be attained in the diet
- Each vitamin may contribute to numerous reactions and serve multiple roles within the body
- **Water-soluble vitamins:**
    - **Vitamin C, B_1, B_2, B_3, B_6, pantothenic acid,** and **biotin** are all involved in mitochondrial energy metabolism
    - **Folic acid** and **vitamin B_{12}** are mainly involved in nucleic acid synthesis (production of cells such as red blood cells, immune cells, and gut mucosa)
    - Vitamin C also serves as an **antioxidant**
        - Antioxidants protect against the damaging effects of **free radicals** – molecules that have at least one unpaired electron which can cause oxidative damage to many components of the body
- **Fat-soluble vitamins:**
    - **Vitamin A** and **E** have antioxidant properties
    - **Vitamin A** also forms the visual pigments of the eye; is particularly important for night vision, but also normal vision
    - **Vitamin D** promotes calcium absorption and bone formation
    - **Vitamin K** is necessary for proper blood-clotting

Learn More: Sport Nutrition Textbook pgs 222-224

VITAMIN INTAKE FOR ATHLETES

- Data used to develop RDA values did not usually include athletes; may not be accurate for evaluating the nutritional needs of those engaged in regular strenuous exercise

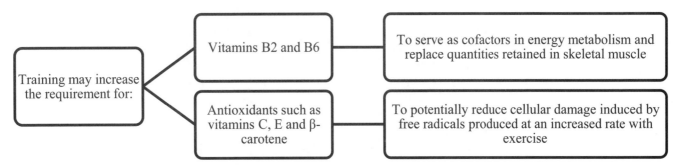

- These elevated needs can be met by consuming a balanced high-CHO, moderate-protein, low-fat diet where energy intake matches energy requirements of training

Learn More: Sport Nutrition Textbook pgs 225-226

MACROMINERALS AND MICROMINERALS

- In nutrition, the term mineral usually refers to the dietary constituents essential to life processes
- Essential minerals are categorized as either macrominerals or microminerals (trace elements)
- At least 20 macrominerals and 14 trace elements have been identified as essential for maintenance of health
    - Macrominerals are present in relatively large quantities
    - Microminerals constitute less than 0.01% of total body mass and are therefore needed in quantities of less than 100 mg/day
- **Major macrominerals**
    - **Calcium** and **phosphorus** are building blocks for body tissues such as bones
    - **Sodium**, **potassium**, and **chlorine** serve as electrolytes
    - **Magnesium** is essential for normal function of enzymes involved in energy metabolism
    - **Sulfur** helps to maintains acid-base balance
- **Major microminerals**
    - **Zinc** and **copper** are essential for normal function of enzymes involved in energy metabolism; zinc also regulates immune function
    - **Iron** transports O_2 and regulates immune function
    - **Chromium** and **iodine** regulate hormone actions and production
    - **Manganese**, **molybdenum**, and **selenium** form cofactors for energy metabolism
    - **Fluorine** promotes bone and teeth formation
    - **Cobalt** is needed for development of red blood cell production
- Trace amounts of arsenic, nickel, silicon, tin, and vanadium may also be essential, but deficiencies or excesses are extremely rare

Learn More: Sport Nutrition Textbook pgs 226-229

ISSUES RELATED TO INADEQUATE MINERAL INTAKE

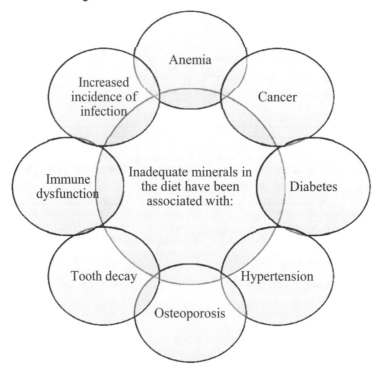

Inside the central circle: Inadequate minerals in the diet have been associated with:

Surrounding circles: Anemia, Cancer, Diabetes, Hypertension, Osteoporosis, Tooth decay, Immune dysfunction, Increased incidence of infection

Learn More: Sport Nutrition Textbook pg 226

RISK FACTORS FOR INADEQUATE MINERAL INTAKE AMONG ATHLETES

- Major risk factors for mineral deficiency among athletes:
  1. **The demand to maintain a low body weight** – usually achieved with chronic low energy intake
     - At risk: gymnasts, jockeys, ballet dancers
  2. **The demand to make competition weight** – usually involves drastic weight-loss regimens to make desired weight category
     - At risk: weight class sports such as rowing, wrestling, boxing, judo
  3. **The demand for very low body fat** – usually involves drastic weight-loss regimens to achieve maximal results
     - At risk: bodybuilders
  4. **Vegetarian diets** – endurance athletes may have difficulty attaining adequate calories and nutrients needed for training
  5. **Training in hot, humid environments** – endurance athletes have significant losses in sweat

Learn More: Sport Nutrition Textbook pg 232

MICRONUTRIENTS AS THE BUILDING BLOCKS OF TISSUES

- **Calcium** and **phosphorus** are structural components of bones and teeth
  - o Bone undergoes continuous turnover and remodeling of its mineral and collagen matrix with simultaneous release and uptake of calcium
  - o The hormones **calcitonin** and **parathyroid hormone (PTH)** are principally involved in the regulation of bone maintenance and metabolism
    - PTH stimulates bone demineralization when calcium levels in circulation are low
    - PTH and ultraviolet radiation from sunlight also stimulate production of vitamin D in the skin which promotes uptake of calcium in the small intestine
    - Calcitonin is released from the thyroid gland and stimulates bone formation when plasma calcium rises
  - o Inadequate calcium intake and consequent lack of bone maintenance leads to **osteoporosis**
  - o Phosphorus deficiency is rare as many foods contain substantial quantities

Learn More: Sport Nutrition Textbook pgs 230-232

MICRONUTRIENT DEFICIENCY AND OSTEOPOROSIS

- Risk of osteoporosis can be reduced by maximizing calcium storage at an early age and minimizing calcium loss; **intake of 1,000 -1,300 mg/day is recommended**
  - o Risk factors for osteoporosis:
    1. Inadequate calcium intake
    2. Low estrogen levels
    3. Alcohol and caffeine intake
    4. Family history
    5. Female gender
    6. Amount and type of physical activity – weight-bearing activities promote the deposition of calcium in bone
- **Amenorrhea** (absence of menstruation) is associated with a high risk of osteoporosis due to chronically low estrogen levels; usually caused by low energy intake and high physical activity with the presence of very low body fat – **calcium supplementation is recommended**
  - o Amenorrhea in young athletes may hinder bone growth when it should be forming at its maximum rate – increasing consumption of calcium to 120% of the RDA is warranted
- **Vitamin D** – required for normal absorption of dietary calcium; deficiency is associated with brittle bones
- **Vitamin C** – required for normal production of collagen; important for the maintenance of connective tissue and cartilage
- **Fluorine** – necessary for normal formation of healthy bones and teeth, as well as protection against dental caries (tooth decay by oral bacteria)

Learn More: Sport Nutrition Textbook pgs 230-231

MICRONUTRIENTS AS ANTIOXIDANTS

- Vitamin C, E, and β-carotene (derived from vitamin A) have antioxidant properties; selenium, copper, and manganese are components of antioxidant enzymes involved in the defense against free radicals
- Vitamin antioxidants prevent or limit the potentially damaging actions of free radicals by converting them into less reactive compounds
- Athletes may need slightly greater quantities due to exercise-induced increases in free-radical formation and lipid peroxidation (abstraction of reactive H+ from fatty acid chains)
- Free radicals can produce forms of damage to cellular membranes, proteins, and DNA
    - Damage to DNA can result in mutations that cause cancer

Learn More: Sport Nutrition Textbook pg 232

EXERCISE-INDUCED FREE RADICALS AND REACTIVE OXYGEN SPECIES

- Damaged muscle provokes an immune response – white blood cells (WBC) are attracted to the tissue to begin breaking down damaged fibers and initiate repair
- Repair process involves the production of free-radical **reactive oxygen species (ROS)** which can cause oxidative damage and are believed to be an underlying cause of disrupted muscle homeostasis and muscle soreness
- Unaccustomed muscle actions and eccentric contractions (in particular) can cause significant damage to myofibers and consequently promote homeostasis-disrupting free-radical damage.

> **Performance-related effects of exercise-induced muscle damage**
>
> - Muscle pain, soreness, and stiffness
> - Reduced range of motion
> - Higher than normal blood lactate concentration
> - Higher perceived exertion during exercise
> - Loss of strength and dynamic power output that can last from 5-10 days
> - Impaired restoration of muscle glycogen due to impaired ability to take up glucose from blood – decreased endurance in subsequent exercise bouts

- Free radicals and ROS are also produced during the aerobic processes of cellular metabolism in the mitochondria (metabolism of O_2)
- Additional sources of ROS and free radicals include:
    - Ultraviolet light (UV rays)
    - Cigarette smoke
    - Alcohol
    - High-fat diets (enhanced lipid peroxidation)
    - Metabolic actions of WBCs that occur during the eradication of foreign materials or bacteria

Learn More: Sport Nutrition Textbook pg 233

FREE RADICALS AND POTENTIAL FOR ADAPTATION

- Free radicals and ROS can cause deleterious effects on muscle function and cellular homeostasis when produced in excess without counter-effective antioxidant action; however, it is now understood that they are generated in a controlled manner by skeletal muscle in response to physiological stimuli and play important roles in adaptations of muscle relative to the stress encountered
    - Includes optimization of contractile performance and changes in gene expression
- **What is the practical application?** – Major doses of supplemental antioxidants may potentially negate training adaptations by thwarting free radical and ROS dynamics related to adaptation

Learn More: Sport Nutrition Textbook pg 233-235

ANTIOXIDANT PROTECTION

- Antioxidants prevent ROS oxidation through the following mechanisms:
    1. Prevention of ROS formation
    2. Interception of ROS attack by scavenging reactive metabolites and converting them into less reactive molecules
    3. Binding to transition metal ion catalysts, such as copper and iron, to prevent initiation of free-radical reactions
    4. Reaction with free radicals to prevent continued lipid peroxidation
    5. Provision of a favorable environment for the effective functioning of other antioxidants or production of new antioxidants

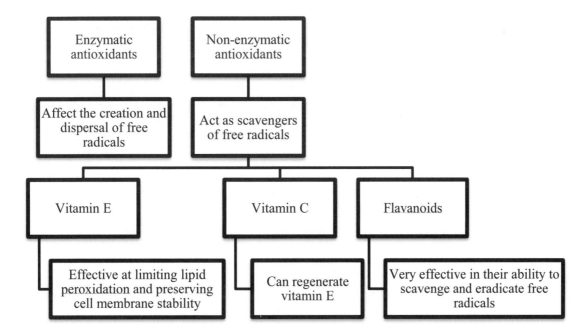

Learn More: Sport Nutrition Textbook pgs 235-236

HIGH-DOSE ANTIOXIDANT SUPPLEMENTATION

- Antioxidants protect against ROS-induced cellular damage, but high-dose supplementation is not advised
  - Increased intake of vitamin E and β-carotene among smokers can actually increase the risk of lung cancer
    - Excess antioxidant action can interfere with important processes needed to break down damaged/hazardous cells in the body (e.g., the killing of cancer cells)
  - Large doses of vitamin C are associated with urinary stone formation, impaired copper absorption, and diarrhea
  - Large doses of vitamin A consumed by pregnant women can cause birth defects
  - Large doses of vitamin E can impair absorption of vitamins A and K
- **Take Home Message: more is not always better**

Learn More: Sport Nutrition Textbook pgs 238-239

ANTIOXIDANT SUPPLEMENTATION CONSIDERATIONS FOR ATHLETES

- More research is needed to document the effects of long-term antioxidant use, but the following facts may help athletes decide whether to supplement or not:
  1. Numerous studies indicate that the body's natural antioxidant defense system is enhanced as an adaptation to exercise
  2. Supplementation does not directly improve exercise performance; recent studies indicate that it may impair the adaptive response to exercise training
  3. Individuals who exercise regularly have a lower incidence of CHD, obesity, diabetes, and some types of cancer compared to sedentary people, suggesting that the benefits of regular exercise outweigh the risks of free-radical-mediated damage
  4. Mega-doses of antioxidant vitamins can have undesirable side effects in some individuals
  5. Athletes can obtain sufficient intakes of natural antioxidants by consuming a well-balanced diet rich in a variety of fruits and vegetables

Learn More: Sport Nutrition Textbook pg 239

IRON INTAKE AND IRON-DEFICIENCY ANEMIA

- **Iron** – essential for oxidative metabolism and O_2 transport; found in hemoglobin, myoglobin, and body storage
- RDA – 8 mg for male; 18 mg for females
- Adult male storage = about 1,000 mg, adult female storage = 300-500 mg, 18-21 year-old female storage = < 200 mg; storage is virtually absent in adolescents
  - Female and adolescent athletes are at a higher risk for iron-deficiency anemia
- Gradual depletion of storage iron is referred to as iron drain: **normal iron status → iron depletion → iron deficiency → iron deficiency anemia**

- Major causes of iron-deficiency anemia among athletes:
  o Low energy intake
  o Insufficient iron intake to maintain stores
  o Low meat consumption

Learn More: Sport Nutrition Textbook pgs 239-242

NEGATIVE EFFECTS OF IRON-DEFICIENCY ANEMIA

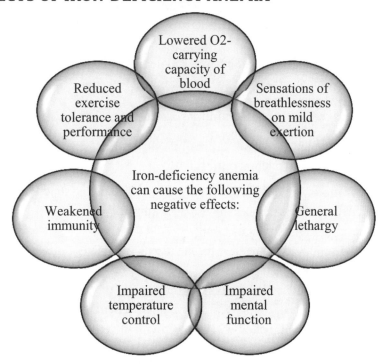

- Anemia (lack of healthy red blood cells) can also arise from deficiencies of vitamin B_6, vitamin B_{12}, folic acid, and copper

Learn More: Sport Nutrition Textbook pgs 239-242

EXERCISE AND IRON INTAKE

- Iron requirements among athletes can be higher due to the following actions that may induce losses up to 70% greater when compared to sedentary individuals
  o Hemolysis of red blood cells
  o Alterations in iron metabolism
  o Increased iron loss in sweat and urine
  o Increased red blood cell production and myoglobin content in muscle (endurance and altitude training)

- Considerations for adequate iron intake and absorption:
  - Heme iron found in animal tissues is absorbed more effectively than nonheme iron (10%-30% compared to 2%-10%)
  - Vitamin C facilitates nonheme iron absorption (e.g., tomatoes added to a spinach salad triples absorption)
  - Tannins in tea, phosphates, and excessive fiber may decrease the bioavailability of nonheme iron
  - Individuals with greater storage have greater absorption capabilities
  - Vegetarians usually encounter few high-absorption iron sources in the diet; these individuals should choose green leafy vegetables, legumes, iron-fortified breads and cereals, and pasta as mainstay foods
- Mega-doses are not advised (toxicity); routine iron supplementation should not be employed without medical supervision following the diagnosis of iron-deficiency anemia

Learn More: Sport Nutrition Textbook pgs 240-242

MICRONUTRIENTS AND IMMUNE FUNCTION

- Heavy exercise and nutrition can both independently influence immune function, but influence is greatest when strenuous exercise is combined with poor nutrition
- Key micronutrients specific to immune function:
  - Vitamin B_{12} and folic acid are needed for the normal production of white blood cells and defend the body against invading pathogens
  - Vitamins A, C and E are needed for normal functioning of immune defense cells
  - Minerals such as zinc, iron, copper and selenium are essential for optimal immune function
- The role of nutrients and immune function will be dealt with in detail in Chapter 16

Learn More: Sport Nutrition Textbook pg 244

MICRONUTRIENTS AS ELECTROLYTES

- Electrolytes conduct electric currents (e.g., nerve impulses) when dissolved in water
- Major electrolytes in the body – sodium, potassium, chloride, bicarbonate, phosphate, sulfate, magnesium, calcium
- Sodium, chloride, and potassium serve to maintain intra- as well as extra-cellular fluid balance and resting cell membrane charge differential (e.g., resting membrane potential, -70 mV); when altered cellular excitation can occur
- **Sodium** – maintains normal body fluid balance, osmotic pressure, and blood pressure; normal fluid levels are critical for nerve impulse transmission and muscle contraction
  - Estimated minimum requirement in adults is 500 mg/day, adequate intake is 1,500 mg/day, upper recommended intake is 2,400 mg/day; **average US intake is reported to exceed 4,500 mg/day** – known to negatively affect blood pressure
  - Excess intake reflects consumption of processed foods (salt is a cheap preservative) and addition of table salt to meals

- o   Low blood sodium (hyponatremia) can occur with prolonged sweating or excessive consumption of water over a period of several hours
- **Chloride** – commonly consumed as sodium-chloride; serves the same purposes as sodium and assists in the formation of hydrochloric acid in the stomach
    - o   Due to the relationship requirements closely parallel sodium
- **Potassium** – serves to regulate body fluid homeostasis and the generation of electrical impulses in nerves, skeletal muscle, and the heart
    - o   Estimated minimum requirement in adults is 2,000 mg/day, adequate intake is 4,700 mg/day
    - o   Low blood potassium levels (hypokalemia) are rare but have been reported in persons suffering from recurring diarrhea and after prolonged diuretic administration

Learn More: Sport Nutrition Textbook pgs 245-246

CLOSER LOOK AT OTHER KEY MICRONUTRIENT FUNCTIONS

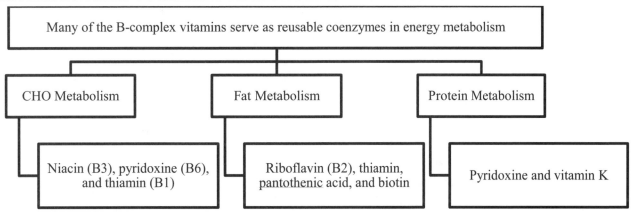

- Zinc serves either a structural or catalytic role in more than 200 functions involved in energy metabolism, normal cell replication, immune function and wound healing; plays a role in appetite regulation
    - o   RDA 11 mg/day for males; 8 mg/day for females
    - o   Prolonged exercise may cause significant losses in sweat and urine, but no evidence has proven this causes a need for supplementation
- Magnesium is an essential factor for more than 300 enzymatic actions during processes such as muscle contraction, glycogen breakdown, protein synthesis, nerve transduction, and fat oxidation
    - o   RDA 420 mg/day for males; 320 mg/day for females
    - o   Losses occur in sweat and urine; a period of heavy training could induce a state of mild deficiency, particularly when training in warm environments
- Copper is a cofactor of various enzymes; appears to be needed for the proper use of iron; plays a role in energy metabolism, synthesis of hemoglobin, hormones, and connective tissue
    - o   RDA 0.9 mg/day for males and females

Learn More: Sport Nutrition Textbook pgs 242-244, 246-247

MICRONUTRIENT STATUS AMONG ATHLETES

- A diagnosis of vitamin or mineral deficiency is best made by considering a variety of data sources:
  - o Blood analysis
  - o Assessment of dietary intake
  - o Clinical symptoms
- **Vitamin considerations for elite athletes**
  - o Ideally, athletes should obtain all of their nutrients from food
  - o A well-balanced diet containing foods from each of the five food groups (meat, dairy, cereal, fruit, and vegetables) should provide adequate amounts of all 13 essential vitamins
  - o Female adolescent athletes and athletes attempting to maintain a low body weight are at the greatest risk for deficiency
- **Mineral considerations for elite athletes**
  - o The assessment of adequate mineral and trace element intake is difficult due to multiple factors:
    - Differences in bioavailability (depending on chemical form) among various food sources
    - Not all foods have been properly analyzed for their mineral content
    - Plasma concentrations do not accurately reflect storage
  - o Data does suggest that iron, zinc, calcium and magnesium status may be of some concern, particularly with younger athletes and female athletes of all ages

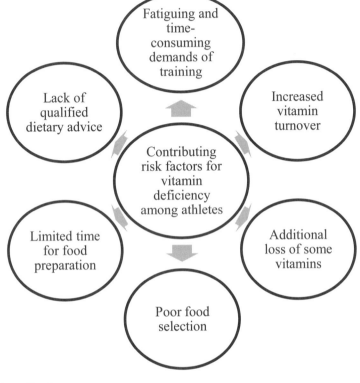

Learn More: Sport Nutrition Textbook pgs 248-251

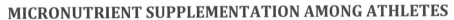

MICRONUTRIENT SUPPLEMENTATION AMONG ATHLETES

- Current research demonstrates that excess vitamin or mineral intake does not enhance performance unless the athlete is currently deficient or follows a very low-calorie diet
- Mineral compounds considered to have ergogenic effects:
  - o Phosphate salts are suggested to increase the re-synthesis of ATP for energy
  - o Bicarbonate (consumed as sodium bicarbonate) has been shown to improve performance during events in which lactic acid accumulation is a major cause of fatigue (e.g., 400m running), but the 20 g needed to be effective commonly causes gastrointestinal discomfort and diarrhea

Learn More: Sport Nutrition Textbook pgs 251-252

SUMMARY MICRONUTRIENT INTAKE CONSIDERATIONS FOR ATHLETES

- Supplementation of micronutrients or antioxidants is only necessary for at-risk individuals; within any group, mega-doses usually do more harm than good
  - Most vitamins function mainly as coenzymes in the body; after these systems are saturated, the vitamin in free form can become toxic
- Specific nutrient recommendations may be useful for athlete groups that are at risk for marginal mineral intake, such as:
  - Those who compete in events in which low body weight is essential for success
  - Those who compete within certain body-weight categories
  - Those who engage in prolonged training in hot and humid environments
  - Vegetarians
- Recommendations to ensure adequate calcium when on an energy-restricted diet:
  - Include three servings per day of low-fat dairy foods
  - Include these dairy foods in high-CHO meals (e.g., skim milk and cereal)
  - Eat fish with bones (e.g., sardines)
  - Include calcium-enriched soy products
  - Eat green leafy vegetables
- Recommendations to ensure adequate iron intake in a high-CHO diet:
  - Eat foods rich in heme iron at least four times a week
  - Eat iron-fortified foods (e.g., breakfast cereal)
  - Include nonheme iron food sources frequently (e.g., legumes, green leafy vegetables)
  - Combine nonheme iron foods with meat or foods rich in vitamin C to increase iron absorption
  - Avoid drinking tea at meals
- It is recommended that amenorrheic female athletes are recommended take a calcium supplement

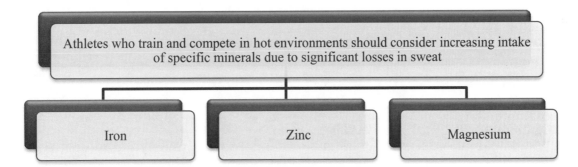

Summary Concept:

- A well-balanced diet can easily correct micronutrient deficiencies, with the possible exceptions of iron and calcium shortfalls

Learn More: Sport Nutrition Textbook pgs 252-253

• REVIEW YOUR KNOWLEDGE

Match the Following Terms

1.____ Free radicals		a. Can occur with inadequate calcium intake
2.____ Electrolytes		b. Lack of healthy red blood cells
3.____ Lipid peroxidation		c. Low blood potassium
4.____ Copper		d. Facilitates nonheme iron absorption
5.____ Parathyroid hormone		e. Suggested to improve ATP re-synthesis
6.____ Hypokalemia		f. Function to conduct nerve impulses
7.____ Osteoporosis		g. Process involving the abstraction of reactive H^+ from FA chains
8.____ Phosphate salts		h. Appears to be needed for the proper use of iron
9.____ Vitamin C		i. Contain unpaired electrons that cause oxidative damage
10.____ Anemia		j. Stimulates bone demineralization

Knowledge and Competency Exercises

11. _____ promotes calcium absorption and bone formation; deficiency is associated with brittle bones.

12. True or False *(circle one)* There are 13 different essential vitamins, including 4 fat-soluble and 9 water-soluble compounds.

13. List three vitamins for which training may increase the daily requirement.

a) _____   b) _____   c) _____

14. Trace elements constitute less than 0.01% of total body mass and are therefore needed in daily quantities of
_____.

15. List five issues or diseases associated with inadequate minerals in the diet.

a) _____

b) _____

c) _____

d) _____

e) _____

16. Complete the following table related to risk factors for marginal mineral intake among athletes.

Conditions and causes	At-risk athletes
The demand to maintain a low body weight	
The demand to make competition weight	
The demand for very low body fat	
Vegetarian diets	
Training in hot, humid conditions	

17. True or False *(circle one)* Alcohol and caffeine intake are considered risk factors for the development of osteoporosis.

18. List four negative effects on performance caused by exercise-induced muscle damage.

a) _____

b) _____

c) _____

d) _____

19. True or False *(circle one)* Free radicals are generated in a controlled manner in response to physiological stress and may play important roles in muscle adaptation.

20. True or False *(circle one)* Large doses of vitamin C ingested by pregnant women are known to cause birth defects.

21. _____ and _____ athletes are at the highest risk for iron-deficiency anemia.

22. List four negative effects associated with iron-deficiency anemia.

a) _____

b) _____

c) _____

d) _____

23. True or False *(circle one)* The average intake of sodium in the US is reported to be three times greater than the adequate intake value set for the mineral.

24. List five contributing risk factors for vitamin deficiency among elite athletes.

a) _____

b) _____

c) _____

d) _____

e) _____

25. True or False *(circle one)* Current research demonstrates that excess vitamin or mineral intake does not enhance performance unless the athlete is currently deficient or follows a very low-calorie diet.

• ASSESS YOUR KNOWLEDGE

1. Which of the following vitamins can protect against the potentially damaging effects of free radicals in the body?

    a.   Vitamin B_{12}
    b.   Vitamin K
    c.   Cobalt
    d.   Vitamin A

2. An athlete with amenorrhea should supplement which of the following?

    a.   Zinc
    b.   Magnesium
    c.   Calcium
    d.   Vitamin C

3. Which of the following statements concerning antioxidants is <u>INCORRECT</u>?

    a.   The body's natural antioxidant system is enhanced as an adaptation to exercise
    b.   Individuals who exercise regularly have a lower incidence of disease, suggesting the benefits of regular exercise outweigh the risk of free-radical-mediated damage
    c.   Large supplemental doses of antioxidants may be beneficial for athletes who train vigorously
    d.   Athletes can obtain sufficient intake of natural antioxidants by consuming a balanced diet rich in a variety of fruits and vegetables

4. Which of the following selections represents the average absorption range for iron in nonheme food sources?

    a.   2% - 10%
    b.   5% - 15%
    c.   8% - 20%
    d.   10% - 30%

5. Which of the following electrolytes ingested in excess can have a negative effect on blood pressure?

    a.   Potassium
    b.   Sulfate
    c.   Sodium
    d.   Magnesium

6. Which of the following athlete groups are at the greatest risk for vitamin deficiency?

    a. Male high school wrestler
    b. Female Olympic sprinters
    c. Female adolescent gymnasts
    d. Male college baseball players

7. Which of the following micronutrients has been shown to improve performance in events in which lactic acid accumulation is a major cause of fatigue?

    a. Iron
    b. Vitamin B$_{12}$
    c. Phosphate
    d. Sodium bicarbonate

8. Athletes who train in hot environments should consider increasing their intake of which of the following minerals due to significant losses that can occur during sweating?

    a. Calcium
    b. Magnesium
    c. Chromium
    d. Fluorine

9. Which of the following micronutrients is essential for oxygen transport?

    a. Folic acid
    b. Iodine
    c. Iron
    d. Chlorine

10. Which of the following does not contribute to reactive oxygen species production which can cause oxidative cellular damage throughout the body?

    a. High-protein diets
    b. Aerobic processes of cellular metabolism within the mitochondria
    c. Cigarette smoke
    d. Metabolic actions of white blood cells that occur during the eradication of foreign materials or bacteria

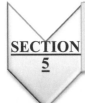

• CHECK YOUR WORK

SPORT NUTRITION CHAPTER 10 ANSWERS

Match the Following Terms

1. I

2. F

3. G

4. H

5. J

6. C

7. A

8. E

9. D

10. B

Knowledge and Competency Exercises

11. Vitamin D

12. True

13. **Possible answers include**: Vitamins B_2, B_6, C, E, and β-carotene

14. Less than 100 mg

15. **Possible answers include**: anemia, cancer, diabetes, hypertension, osteoporosis, tooth decay, immune dysfunction, and increased incidence of infection

16.

Conditions and causes	At risk athletes
The demand to maintain a low body weight	*Gymnasts, jockeys, ballet dancers*
The demand to make competition weight	*Weight class sports, wrestling, boxing, judo*
The demand for very low body fat	*Bodybuilders*
Vegetarian diets	*Endurance athletes*
Training in hot, humid conditions	*Endurance athletes*

17. True

18. **Possible answers include:** muscle pain, soreness, and stiffness, reduced range of motion, higher than normal blood lactate concentration, higher perceived exertion during exercise, loss of strength and dynamic power output that can last from 5-10 days, impaired restoration of muscle glycogen due to impaired ability to take up glucose from blood

19. True

20. False

21. Female, adolescent

22. **Possible answers include:** Lowered O_2-carrying capacity of blood, sensations of breathlessness on mild exertion, general lethargy, impaired mental function, impaired temperature control, weakened immunity, reduced exercise tolerance and performance

23. True

24. **Possible answers include:** Fatiguing and time-consuming demands of training, increased vitamin turnover, additional loss of some vitamins, poor food selection, limited time for food preparation, lack of qualified dietary advice

25. True

Assess Your Knowledge

1. D

2. C

3. C

4. A

5. C

6. C

7. D

8. B

9. C

10. A

SECTION 1

• LEARNING GOALS

Upon completing this section, along with its corresponding chapter, you should understand the following:

1. The definition of a dietary or nutritional supplement

2. The issues with purported claims of popular supplements

3. How to evaluate and critically examine nutrition supplement research to discern if the product has truly been shown to be useful

4. Relevant information and purported claims related to dietary supplements that have not been clearly proven to provide ergogenic effects

5. Relevant information and purported claims related to dietary supplements that may work but require more research to make definitive conclusions

6. The mechanisms of action, ergogenic effects, and potential side effects of dietary supplements that have been proven to improve sport performance

7. The potential dangers of contaminated nutritional supplements on the market that can result in a positive drug test among athletes

8. The ingredients identified in supplements that are banned by the IOC or can cause a positive doping outcome in some athletes

NUTRITIONAL SUPPLEMENTATION

- Nutritional (dietary) supplements
  - Use is not a novel concept; dietary methods for improving performance were documented as early as 500 BC
  - Taken as **ergogenic aids** – nutrient or external factor used to improve performance
  - Should not be used as a substitute for food; primarily designed to supplement a deficiency
  - Are believed to be used by 40% - 100% of athletes in one form or another
- From a regulatory standpoint, dietary supplements are treated as nutritional products and are defined as:
  - "Vitamins, minerals, herbs and botanicals, amino acids, and other dietary substances intended to supplement the diet by increasing total dietary intake, or as any concentrate, metabolite, constituent, or combination of these ingredients"

Learn More: Sport Nutrition Textbook pgs 258-259

NONREGULATION OF NUTRITIONAL SUPPLEMENTS

- Many nutritional supplement claims:
  - Are not backed by validated scientific study (studies used are often from non-peer-reviewed journals or independent research)
  - Portray research findings in a way that makes the product appear effective when the findings do not necessarily apply to the population that will use it
  - Declare unrealistic effects or benefits
  - Are difficult to regulate due to minimal US Food and Drug Administration (FDA) oversight within the industry
    - The FDA does not apply any strict regulations to testing, advertising, or promotion
- **Few nutrition supplements have proven benefits related to performance, recovery, or effects on body weight or composition**

Learn More: Sport Nutrition Textbook pgs 258-259

EVALUATING SUPPLEMENT STUDIES

- Buyer Beware Market – Individuals must critically examine claims made within the dietary supplements industry, including the "scientific evidence" that supports the claims

- The following are factors to consider when evaluating the claims and research behind supplements purported to be ergogenic aids:
    - Does the study have a clear, specific hypothesis?
        - Some studies use a "shotgun" approach
    - Was the study implemented on cells, muscle, animals or humans?
        - Test tube samples are not exposed to the same physiological dynamics as a full living organism
        - There are many known differences between rats and humans
    - Is the population for which claims are applied identical to the population examined in the study?
        - Nutritional supplements may help an individual with a specific deficiency or disease, but this is rarely applicable to healthy athletes
    - Were external variables controlled?
        - Conditions should be the same within all trials and groups
    - Was the study placebo controlled?
    - Were adequate techniques used?
    - Were the trials randomized?
        - Randomization reduces the confounding effects of variables that were not controlled
    - Was a crossover design used?
        - Crossover design allows the same subjects to perform a placebo and treatment trial
    - Was participant assignment random?
    - Do other studies confirm the findings?
    - Was the study peer-reviewed?
- After considering all of the factors, it is easy to see why many purported claims do not truly reflect the ergogenic potential of the product

Learn More: Sport Nutrition Textbook pgs 259-260

SUPPLEMENTS PURPORTED TO BE ERGOGENIC AIDS

- **Androstenedione**
    - Synthetic product believed to stimulate endogenous testosterone synthesis, increase muscle mass and improve recovery
    - Found to not increase testosterone or have any effect on strength; one study reported a decrease in healthy, HDL cholesterol
    - Increases risk of estrogen production in males
    - Substance is banned by the International Olympic Committee (IOC)
- **Bee Pollen**
    - Includes bee saliva, plant nectar, and pollen containing a mixture of vitamins, minerals, and amino acids
    - Claimed to increase energy levels, enhance physical fitness, improve endurance, boost immune function, aid in weight control, increase longevity, reduce free radical damage, and prevent asthma

- o No data exists to prove its effectiveness as an ergogenic aid or other; research shows no effect on O_2 uptake, exercise performance, or metabolism
- o Can be harmful for people who are allergic to pollens
- **Beta-hydroxy beta methylbutyrate (HMB)**
  - o Metabolite of the essential amino acid leucine; purported to decrease protein breakdown, improve muscle mass gains, recovery and immune function as well as increase strength
  - o Studies related to performance reveal conflicting results; some show increases in lean mass and strength while others have demonstrated no effects
  - o Recent compelling evidence related to clinical muscle wasting conditions shows that HMB may be beneficial
    - ▪ HMB seems to reduce the breakdown of muscle protein by inhibiting pathways of protein metabolism and stimulating protein synthesis
  - o HMB may function as an ergogenic aid, but users should note that most studies used 3 g/day, whereas most recovery products currently on the market contain extremely small quantities
- **Boron**
  - o Trace element which influences calcium and magnesium metabolism, steroid hormone metabolism, and membrane function
  - o Present in vegetables and non-citrus fruits
  - o Claimed to improve bone density, muscle mass, and strength
  - o Found to increase bone mineral density in postmenopausal women who were deprived of boron for 4 months, but had no effect on bone density, muscle mass, or strength among men
  - o Does not appear to be an effective ergogenic aid for healthy adults
- **L-Carnitine**
  - o Vitamin-like substance important for FA transport; purported to improve fat oxidation and weight loss, reduce lactate production, and improve VO_2max
  - o Is derived from red meats and dairy products in the diet and from production within the body
  - o Generally marketed as a "fat burner" or to improve "sharpness"
  - o Became popular after rumors that it helped the Italian national soccer team to become world champions in 1982

Sources of Dietary Carnitine

Source	Total L-carnitine content (mg/100g)
Sheep	210
Lamb	78
Beef	64
Pork	30
Rabbit	21
Chicken	7.5
Milk	2.0
Egg	0.8
Peanut	0.1

  - o Numerous studies found supplemental L-carnitine did not enhance muscle L-carnitine levels due to low bioavailability and transport into the muscle; it seems that when adequate levels exist in the muscle, additional dietary L-carnitine will not improve concentrations
  - o In a novel study, enhancing insulin action through a carbohydrate feeding promoted uptake, but the feeding (kcal) more than offset the potential for weight loss promoted by enhanced carnitine
- **Choline**
  - o Precursor of the neurotransmitter acetylcholine; purported to improve performance and decrease fatigue

- o Is abundant in meat and dairy products
- o Plasma levels are reduced after strenuous exercise; 40% decrease measured in participants of the 1985 Boston Marathon
- o Supplement claims are based largely on theory and "test tube" studies, interesting finds have occurred during human studies but grounds to classify choline as an ergogenic aid are insufficient

- **Chromium Picolinate**
  - o Trace element that potentiates insulin action; purported to build muscle and aid in weight loss
  - o Present in foods such as brewer's yeast, American cheese, mushrooms and wheat germ; considered an essential nutrient
  - o Currently, no supporting evidence exists that illustrates chromium picolinate to be effective for increasing lean body mass by itself
  - o During laboratory studies using cultured cells, chromium picolinate was demonstrated to accumulate in the cells, causing direct chromosome damage

- **Coenzyme Q10**
  - o High-energy phosphate carrier within the mitochondria important for direct energy production; purported to improve VO_2max and performance, as well as reduce fatigue
  - o Used therapeutically to treat cardiovascular disease and promote recovery from cardiac surgery; improves functional capacity of cardiac rehab patients
  - o No research proves that coenzyme Q10 is effective as an ergogenic aid for healthy adults

- **Fish Oil**
  - o Polyunsaturated fatty acids (PUFAs) purported from an ergogenic standpoint to increase VO_2max
  - o Researchers have suggested that increasing PUFA concentrations in RBC membranes may improve membrane flexibility, resulting in improved peripheral O_2 supply
  - o Has not been proven to be an effective ergogenic aid, but may be used to supplement the diet for health purposes

- **Dehydroepiandrosterone (DHEA)**
  - o Precursor of testosterone and estradiol; claimed to improve immune function, increase lifespan, protect against cardiovascular disease, increase lean body mass, and improve overall well-being
  - o Is a weak androgen steroid hormone synthesized primarily in early adulthood (20-25 years of age) by the adrenal cortex
  - o Often marketed as a super-hormone to slow the aging process, the FDA has little control over these manufacturer claims because the substance occurs naturally
  - o Initial studies examined effects in rats with very promising results – but rats genetically have much lower levels of DHEA when compared to humans
  - o Later human studies have shown minimal benefits for male subjects and negative effects for females
    - A total view of the results is not significantly convincing, but it does seem to indicate that DHEA can have a small effect on muscle mass and immune function in 40-75 year old males
  - o Little is known of its side-effects and potential long-term complications (e.g., simulation of dormant prostate tumors)

- o The IOC has placed it on the banned substances list with zero tolerance
- o The US Senate introduced a bill in 2007 in an attempt to classify DHEA as a controlled substance under the category of anabolic steroids

- **Ginseng**
  - o Root of the *Araliaceous* plant; purported to improve strength, performance, stamina, and cognitive functioning as well as reduce fatigue
  - o Known varieties include American, Chinese, Korean, Japanese, and Siberian
  - o Commonly marketed as an "adaptogen" – a substance that helps the body adapt to stressful situations
  - o Has been used for several thousand years in Asia for its claimed effects of improving sleep, memory, and libido as well as reducing pain associated with heart conditions, headaches, and nausea
  - o Research does not support the purported claims; improvements have been documented with rats, but many of the human studies were poorly designed

- **Medium-Chain Triacylglycerol (MCT)**
  - o Fatty acid chains usually synthesized from coconut oil; purported to supply significant energy, reduces muscle glycogen breakdown, and improve overall performance
  - o Sold as a supplement to replace normal fat due to the belief that they are not stored and can help athletes lose body fat; popular among bodybuilders
  - o Studies show that MCTs do contribute to energy expenditure (3%-7%) when taken with carbohydrates but do not improve exercise performance or time to fatigue
  - o Ingestion of large quantities result in gastrointestinal distress
  - o Does not appear to provide the claimed benefits related to performance

- **Glandulars**
  - o Extracts of animal glands such as the adrenals, the thymus, the pituitary, and the testes; claimed to enhance the function of the equivalent gland in the human body
  - o Claims include improved strength, performance, and stamina
  - o Glandular extracts are metabolized during the digestive process and are inactive when absorbed, making them ineffective as an ergogenic aid

- **Inosine**
  - o Nucleoside purported to increase ATP stores, improve strength, training quality, and overall performance
  - o Supplemental inosine can produce adverse effects in that it increases serum uric acid levels to the degree that it could be associated with gouty arthritis; considered ergolytic (produces effects detrimental to performance)
  - o Inosine supplements should be avoided

- **Lecithin**
  - o A phospholipid that occurs naturally in a variety of food items including beans, eggs and wheat germ; claimed to improve strength and reduce fatigue
  - o It contains both choline and phosphorus; theorized to be an ergogenic aid for this reason
  - o Research has not proven its effectiveness for improving performance

- **Pangamic Acid**

- o Often referred to as vitamin B_{15} but is not a vitamin or essential nutrient and has no known function in the body
- o Claimed to increase O_2 delivery, reduce lactate formation, and improve performance
- o Studies show no positive effects on performance; in contrast, synthetic pangamic acid has been shown to be harmful
- o FDA guidelines forbid its sale as a dietary supplement or drug
- **Phosphate salts (phosphorus)**
  - o Mineral predominantly found in bone; plays an important role in energy metabolism and intracellular buffering
  - o Claimed to increase ATP synthesis, provide energy, and buffer lactic acid with loading
  - o Early studies found an increased VO_2max and decreased lactate concentration among subjects during submaximal cycling and running; many others did not find any benefits
  - o Inconsistencies within study findings and protocol indicates that more research is needed before it can be definitively recommended as an ergogenic aid
- **Phosphatidylserine**
  - o Structural component of cell membranes; usually derived from soy in marketed brands
  - o Claimed to reduce stress responses and improve recovery
  - o A few studies implemented by the same research team seemed to reveal that the compound reduces stress makers of exercise (e.g., cortisol) compared to placebo, but additional research is needed before definite conclusions can be drawn
- **Polylactate**
  - o Polymer of lactate claimed to provide additional energy for optimal performance
  - o Lactate is an important fuel source for the heart and skeletal muscle; polylactate is believed to enhance lactate energy availability when added to a beverage
  - o Has not been found to be an effective ergogenic aid as increases in performance could only occur at ingestion rates that are not tolerated by the gastrointestinal tract
- **Pyruvate and dihydroxyacetone (DHA)**
  - o Intermediates of carbohydrate metabolism formed in the glycolytic pathway; used synergistically as a supplement
  - o Claimed to improve endurance capacity, training recovery, and insulin sensitivity, as well as increase glycogen storage and fat use during exercise
  - o Initial studies with rats seemed to show that pyruvate and DHA accelerated carbohydrate breakdown and produced negative effects on running performance
  - o Later studies with humans showed equivocal results; the studies that revealed positive results were implemented by only one research team, indicating that more research is needed before pyruvate and DHA can be considered ergogenic aids
- **Vanadium**
  - o Trace element purported to aid in weight loss and improve insulin sensitivity
  - o Appears to increase insulin sensitivity in type 2 diabetes patients with insulin resistance but does not seem useful as an ergogenic aid for healthy adults
- **Yohimbine**
  - o α_2-adrenoreceptor blocker purported to increase testosterone, fat-free mass, and strength
  - o No supporting evidence demonstrates its effectiveness as an ergogenic aid

- **Wheat Germ Oil**
  - Extracted from the embryo of wheat; rich in linoleic acid, vitamin E, and octacosanol (an alcohol compound theorized to have ergogenic effects)
  - Advertised to increase endurance, stamina, and vigor
  - Many studies have examined its metabolic effects, but no evidence supports the contention that it is an ergogenic aid

Learn More: Sport Nutrition Textbook pgs 261-291

SUPPLEMENTS CLEARLY PROVEN TO WORK

- **Caffeine** – central nervous system stimulator
- **Creatine** – high energy phosphate carrier
- **Glycerol** – used for training in the heat
- **Sodium bicarbonate** and **sodium citrate** – lactic acid buffers

Learn More: Sport Nutrition Textbook pgs 265-270, 275-281, 283-284, 288, 289-290

CAFFEINE

- Originates naturally in 63 species of plants; main sources include coffee beans, tea leaves, cocoa beans, and cola nuts (coffee accounts for ~75% of all consumption)
- Effects on exercise and cognitive function:
  - **Endurance exercise**
    - Improved endurance capacity with dosages as low as 1.0-3.2 mg/kg of body weight
    - At intensities above 85% VO_2max, 10%-20% improvements in time to exhaustion are typically encountered
    - Caffeine reduces the perceived exertion of any given exercise
  - **Maximal exercise**
    - Generally seems to improve performance during exercise near 100% of VO_2max lasting approximately 5 minutes
    - Improvements suggested to be the effect of caffeine on neuromuscular pathways that facilitate muscle fiber recruitment or increase total fiber recruitment as well as lower perceived exertion
  - **Supramaximal exercise**
    - Appears to have no positive effect on sprint performance; studies that have examined this are limited; therefore, conclusions cannot be definitive
  - **Cognitive functioning**
    - When combined with carbohydrates, caffeine improves concentration, response speed and detection, and performance of complex cognitive tasks during and after exercise
  - **Carbohydrate absorption**
    - Evidence suggests that caffeine enhances ingested carbohydrate absorption, but the optimal dosage is unclear

- **Proven to exert physiological effects that improve performance in most events, lowers the perceived exertion of exercise, and increases cognitive functioning**

Learn More: Sport Nutrition Textbook pgs 265-269

MECHANISMS OF ACTION FOR CAFFEINE

Increases lipolysis and spares muscle glycogen	• Increases circulating epinephrine levels • Influences adenosine receptors that normally inhibit fatty acid oxidation
Increases excitability of muscle fibers	• Has a direct effect on key regulatory enzymes such as phosphorylase • Increases release of calcium from the sarcoplasmic reticulum • Increases the sensitivity of myofilaments to calcium
Influences signals from the brain to motor neurons	• Stimulates neurotransmitter release which may lower perception of effort • May lower the excitation threshold for motor neuron recruitment • Facilitates transmission of nervous signals

Learn More: Sport Nutrition Textbook pgs 269-270

POTENTIAL SIDE EFFECTS OF CAFFEINE

- Side effects caused by stimulation of the central nervous system:
  - Gastrointestinal distress
  - Headaches
  - Tachycardia
  - Restlessness and irritability
  - Tremor
  - Elevated blood pressure
  - Psychomotor agitations
  - Premature left ventricular contractions
- Extremely high intakes have been associated with peptic ulcers, seizures, coma, and even death

Learn More: Sport Nutrition Textbook pg 270

CREATINE

- Naturally occurring compound primarily found in muscle tissue; provides the high-energy phosphate group for ATP regeneration during high-intensity, short duration exercise
- Not an essential nutrient as it is internally synthesized
- Primary dietary sources include fish and red meat, vegetarians consume negligible amounts
- Claimed to improve strength, reduce fatigue, and increase protein synthesis
- Became popular after the 1992 Olympics in Barcelona where multiple gold medal winners used creatine

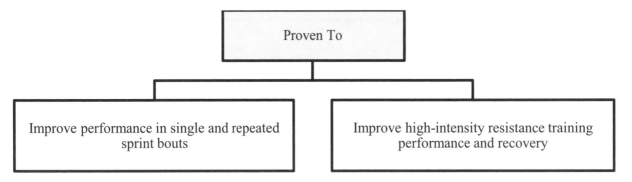

Learn More: Sport Nutrition Textbook pgs 261, 275-276

CREATINE LOADING AND SUPPLEMENTATION

- Loading and daily supplementation:
    - Allows for increased phosphocreatine storage which permits increased work performed during single and repeated bouts of short-term, high-intensity exercise
    - Loading – 20 g/day for 5 days increases total muscle creatine content in men by 20%
    - Subsequent daily doses of 2 g is enough to maintain this concentration
    - Potential weight gain averages about 1 kg; most of the gained mass is suggested to be in the form of cellular water retained in muscle due to an increase in osmolarity

Learn More: Sport Nutrition Textbook pgs 277-278

EFFECTS OF CREATINE ON EXERCISE

- Effects on exercise
    - **High-intensity exercise**
        - Majority of studies show improvements in strength, force production, work until failure, or torque while performing high-intensity repeat sprinting, bench pressing, leg pressing, or cycling

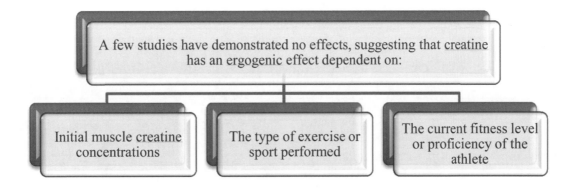

- o **Endurance exercise**
  - ▪ Creatine has no positive effect, and may even be detrimental if weight gain is sufficient to slow down the athlete
- o **Resistance training**
  - ▪ Creatine supplementation augments strength gains by up to 20%-25% depending on many variables
  - ▪ Supplementation allows for more repetitions and thus improved quality of training and anabolic effects
  - ▪ Promotes fluid retention and potential muscle cell swelling which can act as an anabolic signal – potentially increasing protein synthesis
    - • Specific evidence of creatine's influence on protein metabolism has not been found

Learn More: Sport Nutrition Textbook pgs 279-281

MECHANISMS OF ACTION FOR CREATINE

- • Proposed mechanisms of action:
  - o Increased phosphocreatine availability, especially in type II muscle fibers
    - ▪ Evidence indicates that increased stores improve contractile function by maintaining ATP resynthesis
  - o Increased rate of phosphocreatine resynthesis; important for short recovery periods during repeated bouts of maximal exercise
  - o Increased use of phosphocreatine as an energy source could reduce anaerobic glycolysis and lactic acid production, potentially reducing H^+ formation in muscle and delaying fatigue caused by acidity
  - o Could buffer some of the H^+ produced during high-intensity exercise
  - o May have anabolic properties

Learn More: Sport Nutrition Textbook pg 281

SIDE EFFECTS AND SAFETY OF CREATINE

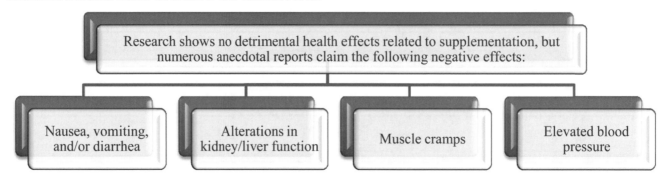

Research shows no detrimental health effects related to supplementation, but numerous anecdotal reports claim the following negative effects:

| Nausea, vomiting, and/or diarrhea | Alterations in kidney/liver function | Muscle cramps | Elevated blood pressure |

Learn More: Sport Nutrition Textbook pg 281

GLYCEROL

- Backbone of a triglyceride molecule
- Initially believed to be a substrate for gluconeogenesis, and therefore able to provide fuel during exercise; research however, has shown that its contribution to fuel supply during exercise is negligible
- Recently found to be an effective supplement for inducing hyperhydration before exercise
  - When ingested with a relatively large volume of water (1 to 2 L), glycerol improves water absorption and increases water retention in the extracellular space, especially in blood plasma
  - Decreases total heat stress as indicated by lower heart rates and temperature
  - Effects on endurance performance remain unclear

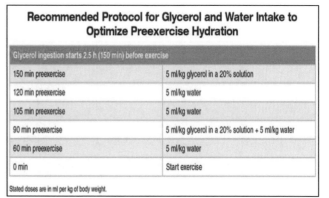

Recommended Protocol for Glycerol and Water Intake to Optimize Preexercise Hydration	
Glycerol ingestion starts 2.5 h (150 min) before exercise	
150 min preexercise	5 ml/kg glycerol in a 20% solution
120 min preexercise	5 ml/kg water
105 min preexercise	5 ml/kg water
90 min preexercise	5 ml/kg glycerol in a 20% solution + 5 ml/kg water
60 min preexercise	5 ml/kg water
0 min	Start exercise
Stated doses are in ml per kg of body weight.	

- Potential mechanisms of action
  - Glycerol may move to the extracellular space and (through osmosis) draw water into this compartment like a sponge
  - A decrease in the plasma osmolarity may increase antidiuretic hormone (ADH) secretion, thus decreasing urine production
- Potential side-effects
  - Nausea
  - Heartache and/or headache
  - Blurred vision
  - Gastrointestinal problems
  - Dizziness
  - Bloating due to the necessity to ingest large quantities of water

Learn More: Sport Nutrition Textbook pgs 283-284

LACTIC ACID BUFFERS

- Sodium bicarbonate
    - Buffer present in blood known as an alkalinizer; functions to reduce acidity in working tissue by buffering H^+ in the blood
    - Many studies provide equivocal results, but it appears to enhance buffering of lactic acid and improve high-intensity exercise performance between approximately 1 and 7 minutes
    - 300 mg/kg of body weight seems to be the optimal dose if side effects are tolerated (bloating, abdominal discomfort, diarrhea)
- Sodium citrate
    - Functions similar to bicarbonate by buffering H+ and limiting the decrease of blood pH
    - Seems to be able to improve high-intensity exercise performance of 2 to 4 minute durations (up to 10 minutes)
    - Typical doses are even higher than sodium bicarbonate at 300-500 mg/kg of body weight with similar potential side-effects

Learn More: Sport Nutrition Textbook pgs 289-290

CONTAMINATION OF NUTRITION SUPPLEMENTS

- Speculation suggests that some of the positive drug tests recently recorded in sport have resulted from the use of nutritional supplements rather than deliberate use of banned products
- The IOC-accredited laboratory in Cologne, Germany recently reported that various steroids (nandrolone being the most prominent) and their precursor compounds were found in a mass-testing of various dietary supplements
    - Of the 634 supplements tested, 94 of them (nearly 15%) contained enough anabolics to cause a positive result on a drug test – none of the products gave any indication on the label that they contained steroids
    - Of supplements made in the United States, almost 20% of the 240 tested contained prohormones
- Ingredients identified in common supplements that are banned by the IOC or can cause a positive doping outcome:
    - Ephedrine
    - Strychnine
    - Androstenedione, andostenediol, DHEA (can lead to elevated testosterone:epitestosterone ratio)
    - 19-norandrostenedione, 19-norandrostenediol, and related compounds (positive test for metabolites of the steroid nandrolone)
- Unfortunately, current legislation does little to protect athletes and other consumers from insufficiently labeled, mislabeled, contaminated, or even unsafe ingredients in dietary supplements
- It is recommended that athletes purchase supplements from reputable brands; contamination is a problem in smaller and more exotic companies, particularly ones that sell steroids or prohormones

Learn More: Sport Nutrition Textbook pgs 291-292

• REVIEW YOUR KNOWLEDGE

Match the Following Terms

1. ____ Boron   a. Must be consumed with relatively large quantities of water to be effective

2. ____ Vanadium   b. Ergogenic benefit claims based on in vitro studies

3. ____ Caffeine   c. Primary dietary sources include red meat and fish

4. ____ Choline   d. α_2-adrenoreceptor blocker purported to increase testosterone

5. ____ HMB   e. Metabolized during digestion and inactive when absorbed

6. ____ Yohimbine   f. Functions to buffer H+ from the blood

7. ____ Creatine   g. Found to increase bone mineral density among postmenopausal women

8. ____ Glycerol   h. Might be useful for clinical muscle wasting conditions

9. ____ Glandulars   i. Appears to be useful for type 2 diabetes

10. ____ Sodium citrate   j. Can reduce the perceived exertion of exercise

Knowledge and Competency Exercises

11. List four factors to consider when evaluating the research claims of a specific supplement.

a) _____

b) _____

c) _____

d) _____

12. True or False? *(circle one)* Few nutrition supplements have proven benefits related to performance, recovery, or effects on body weight or composition.

13. Research has reported a decrease in healthy HDL cholesterol with use of _____.

14. True or False? *(circle one)* Even though inosine has been purported to improve strength, training quality, and overall performance, research has shown it to be a potentially ergolytic compound.

15. _____ is often referred to as vitamin B_{15} but is not a vitamin or essential nutrient, and has no known function in the body.

16. _____ could enhance the availability of an important fuel source for the heart and skeletal muscle but has not been found to be a practical ergogenic aid as increases in performance can only occur at ingestion rates that are not tolerated by the gastrointestinal tract.

17. List three supplements that have been clearly proven in research to be effective ergogenic aids.

a) _____   b) _____   c) _____

18. True or False? *(circle one)* Current legislation does little to protect athletes and other consumers from insufficiently labeled, mislabeled, contaminated, or even unsafe ingredients in dietary supplements.

19. What three factors can influence the ergogenic effectiveness of creatine for a given athlete?

a) _____

b) _____

c) _____

20. List two potential side effects of glycerol supplementation.

a) _____   b) _____

• ASSESS YOUR KNOWLEDGE

1. Which of the following statements related to nutritional supplement claims is INCORRECT?

   a. Many claims are not backed by scientific study
   b. Many claims declare unrealistic effects
   c. Many claims stem from independent research
   d. Many claims are strictly regulated by the FDA through testing

2. Which of the following nutritional supplements claimed to be a useful ergogenic aid simply contains a mixture of vitamins, minerals, and amino acids and has been found to be ineffective?

   a. Carnitine
   b. Fish Oil
   c. Bee pollen
   d. Glandulars

3. Which of the following nutritional supplements has been found to be useful for promoting recovery from cardiac surgery but is not proven to be an effective ergogenic aid for healthy adults?

   a. Coenzyme Q10
   b. Lecithin
   c. Yohimbine
   d. Wheat germ oil

4. Which of the following nutritional supplements is commonly marketed as an "adaptogen" (substance that helps the body deal with stress)?

   a. Pangamic acid
   b. Ginseng
   c. DHA
   d. Creatine

5. Which of the following nutritional supplements is actually a precursor of testosterone and estradiol that is internally synthesized during early adulthood by the adrenal cortex?

   a. Pyruvate
   b. Phosphatidylserine
   c. Glycerol
   d. DHEA

6. Which of the following is <u>not</u> a suggested mechanism of action related to the ergogenic effects of caffeine?

    a. Caffeine increases lipolysis and spares muscle glycogen
    b. Caffeine may increase the excitation threshold for motor neuron recruitment
    c. Caffeine increases excitability of muscle fibers by increasing calcium release from the sarcoplasmic reticulum
    d. Caffeine stimulates the release of catecholamines and other neurotransmitters that could possibly result in decreased perception of effort

7. Which of the following statements related to the ergogenic effects of creatine is INCORRECT?

    a. Creatine supplementation can improve long-distance endurance training by increasing motor unit efficiency
    b. Creatine supplementation can improve force production when performing multiple sets of bench press
    c. Creatine supplementation can improve repeat sprint performance and recovery
    d. Creatine supplementation can allow for additional strength training volume and therefore improved anabolic effects

8. Which of the following describes a potential benefit of glycerol supplementation?

    a. Enhanced buffering of lactic acid
    b. Increased force production
    c. Increased water absorption and retention
    d. Enhanced cognitive functioning

9. Which of the following nutritional supplements might be useful for reducing acidity within working muscle while performing high-intensity exercise for approximately five minutes?

    a. Boron
    b. Androstenedione
    c. Inosine
    d. Sodium bicarbonate

10. Which of the following substances has not been banned by the International Olympic Committee?

    a. Ephedrine
    b. Choline
    c. Strychnine
    d. Androstenedione

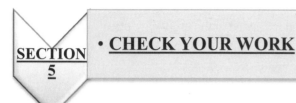

SECTION 5 • **CHECK YOUR WORK**

SPORT NUTRITION CHAPTER 11 ANSWERS

Match the Following Terms

1. G

2. I

3. J

4. B

5. H

6. D

7. C

8. A

9. E

10. F

Knowledge and Competency Exercises

11. **Possible answers:** Does the study have a clear, specific hypothesis? Was the study implemented on cells, muscle, animals or humans? Is the population for which claims are applied identical to the population examined in the study? Were external variables controlled? Was the study placebo controlled? Were adequate techniques used? Were the trials randomized? Was a crossover design used? Was participant assignment random? Do other studies confirm the findings? Was the study peer-reviewed?

12. True

13. Androstenedione

14. True

15. Pangamic Acid

16. Polylactate

17. **Possible answers:** Caffeine, creatine, glycerol, sodium bicarbonate, sodium citrate

18. True

19. **a)** Initial muscle creatine concentrations, **b)** the type of exercise or sport engaged in, **c)** current fitness level and training status of the athlete

20. **Possible answers:** Nausea, heartache and/or headache, blurred vision, gastrointestinal problems, dizziness, bloating due to the necessity to ingest large quantities of water

Assess Your Knowledge

1. D

2. C

3. A

4. B

5. D

6. B

7. A

8. C

9. D

10. B

SECTION 1

• LEARNING GOALS

Upon completing this section, along with its corresponding chapter, you should understand the following:

1. Concepts related to how training adaptations occur with repeated bouts of exercise

2. The adaptations specific to resistance training and endurance training

3. The signals and triggers that occur during exercise that lead to adaptations via protein synthesis

4. The time course of events for adaptation during and after a bout of exercise

5. The effects of nutritional strategies on training adaptations

6. The definitions and potential symptoms of overreaching and overtraining as well as nutritional factors that can increase the risk of developing overtraining syndrome

TRAINING ADAPTATIONS

- Regular physical activity can promote adaptations that result in improved function
- Structured exercise makes use of this principle by planning and systematically applying specific activities at varied training volumes to optimize adaptations and improve performance
- Training adaptations related to endurance and strength training are listed in Table 12.1, pg 296

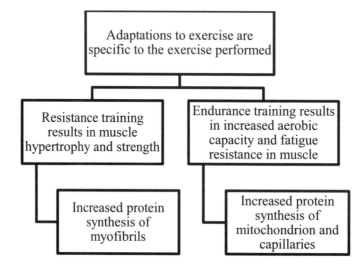

- Growth, metabolism, and creation of new muscle proteins (either myofibril or mitochondrial) depends on signals or factors such as:
  - Nutrient availability
  - pH in the muscle
  - Presence of O_2
  - Presence of reactive oxygen species (ROS)
  - Mechanical stimuli
  - Nervous and endocrine system input
- Training adaptations in skeletal muscle are ultimately generated by the cumulative effects of gene transcription (temporary increases in DNA replication and translation onto new proteins) during recovery periods between bouts of exercise

Learn More: Sport Nutrition Textbook pgs 296-297

SIGNALS AND TRIGGERS FOR EXERCISE-INDUCED ADAPTATIONS

- The complex process of exercise-induced adaptation in skeletal muscle starts with specific molecular events that trigger an increase in protein synthesis
- Those molecular events are initiated during exercise by the following actions:
  - **Changes in muscle stretch or tension**
    - Induces signaling compounds including insulin-like growth factor (IGF) that generate adaptations such as muscle hypertrophy
  - **Changes in intracellular calcium ion concentrations**
    - Elevated concentration in muscle cytoplasm activates calcineurin that acts as a co-regulator of muscle hypertrophy
  - **Changes in the energy charge of a muscle cell**
    - Energy charge is the ratio of ATP and its metabolites (ADP, AMP, P_i) in the cell
      - When ATP is high and metabolites are low, the energy charge is high
      - When ATP is low and metabolites are high, the energy charge is low
      - When the energy charge becomes low the enzyme AMPK becomes active, increasing energy metabolism via glucose uptake and fatty acid breakdown and assisting in cell hypertrophy
  - **Changes in muscle cell energy (redox) potential**
    - Maintenance of energy potential produces free-radical reactive oxygen species (ROS) that aid in adaptations
- The exercise stress itself (along with the previous dynamics) acts on muscle cell DNA through molecular-driven signal pathways that control the following processes:
  - Transcription of genes (specific sequences of DNA) into mRNA (communicates modification of cells)
  - Translation of mRNA into new protein
  - Protein modification that alters catalytic activity (potential for adaptation)
  - Regulation of protein breakdown
  - Regulation of muscle cell division, duplication, and/or synthesis
- **Summary – exercise causes cellular homeostasis disturbances and initiates a cascade of events that ultimately result in an adaptation that will cause less disturbance the next time the same exercise is performed**

Learn More: Sport Nutrition Textbook pgs 297-300

TIME COURSE OF EVENTS FOR ADAPTATION

- The initial responses to exercise usually occur within seconds or minutes (e.g., changes in intracellular calcium)
- The cascade of molecular reactions leading to potential adaptation typically reach maximal activity several hours after exercise
- Gene expression (actions on muscle cell DNA that generate adaptations) seems to peak within 4 to 12 hours after exercise depending on the gene and type of exercise performed
  - Research has shown 4-8 hours after resistance training, 8-12 hours after endurance exercise

- Actual changes in protein synthesis (myofibril or mitochondrial) can begin within hours after exercise but may peak many hours later
    - Studies have shown increased synthesis up to 48 hours after exercise

Learn More: Sport Nutrition Textbook pg 301

NUTRITION EFFECTS ON TRAINING ADAPTATIONS

- Nutrients can have an effect on signaling and therefore regulate or alter training adaptation
- Compounds that can influence training adaptations via nutritional strategies:
    - **The amino acid leucine**
        - BCAAs such as leucine are building blocks and strong signal stimulators for protein synthesis
        - Increased intake alone will not necessarily result in amplified protein synthesis if the other essential amino acids are not available in circulation to serve as building blocks
    - **Muscle glycogen**
        - Research has shown that training with low muscle glycogen can increase gene transcription via reactions such as elevated AMPK due to a low energy charge in the muscle tissue
        - It is unclear if low-glycogen induced reactions result in improvements in performance due to the offsetting factors of lower training intensity and duration potential as well as enhanced physiological stress
    - **Free-radical ROS**
        - Involved in cell-signaling pathways that have been found to be essential for the development of optimal force production (in moderate levels)
        - Supplementation with large doses of antioxidants may interfere with the function of ROS and could therefore reduce training adaptations
    - **Cytokines and other inflammatory markers**
        - Nonsteroidal anti-inflammatory drugs (NSAIDs) such as ibuprofen, aspirin, and naproxen may interfere with the normal inflammatory responses which play a role in adaptations that occur after exercise
        - Some evidence indicates that tissue protein synthesis can be suppressed following high-intensity eccentric exercise as a result of using ibuprofen (1,200 mg)
        - Animal studies have shown that NSAIDs may interfere with muscle regeneration and hypertrophy

Learn More: Sport Nutrition Textbook pgs 302-307

OVERTRAINING AND OVERREACHING

Overreaching
•An accumulation of training and other stresses resulting in a short-term decrement in performance
•Restoration of performance may take **several days to several weeks**

Overtraining
•An accumulation of training and other stresses resulting in a long-term decrement in performance
•Restoration of performance may take **several weeks or months**

- Overreaching and overtraining syndrome can occur when the total of all life stresses exceeds the ability of the body to cope with those stresses
- Proper nutrition can reduce the symptoms of overreaching and reduce the risk of developing overtraining syndrome
- The following nutrition-related factors can increase the risk for overtraining over time by amplifying the physiological stress response of training (i.e., stress hormone reactions):
  - Carbohydrate depletion
    - A high-carbohydrate diet can reduce or delay symptoms of overreaching during prolonged periods of intensified training but not completely prevent them
  - Dehydration
  - Negative energy balance

Potential symptoms of overtraining and overreaching
•Drop in performance
•Washed-out feeling, tired, drained, lack of energy
•Mild leg discomfort, general aches and pains in muscles and joints
•Sleeping problems, insomnia
•Headaches
•Decreased immunity – increased colds or infection
•Decrease in training capacity or intensity, inability to complete training sessions
•Moodiness, irritability, and/or depression
•Loss of enthusiasm for a given sport
•Decreased appetite, eating problems
•Increased incidence of injury
•Reduced maximal lactate and heart rate
•Elevated resting and sleeping heart rate
•No increase in <u>cortisol</u> in response to a stressful bout of exercise

Learn More: Sport Nutrition Textbook pgs 307-310

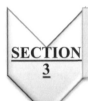

• **REVIEW YOUR KNOWLEDGE**

Match the Following Terms

1. _____ Gene transcription

a. Ratio of ATP and its metabolites (ADP, AMP, Pi) in the cell

2. _____ Energy charge

b. Might interfere with protein synthesis

3. _____ Overreaching

c. Activated by elevated Ca^{2+}

4. _____ NSAIDs

d. DNA replication and translation onto new proteins

5. _____ IGF

e. Short-term decrement in performance capacity

Knowledge and Competency Exercises

6. True or False? *(circle one)* The complex process of exercise-induced adaptation in skeletal muscle starts with specific molecular events that trigger an increase in protein synthesis.

7. List four actions that occur during exercise which can initiate molecular responses that generate adaptations.

a) _____

b) _____

c) _____

d) _____

8. _____ serves to communicate modification of muscle cell function and is therefore translated into newly synthesized proteins to generate adaptation.

9. Gene expression (actions on muscle cell DNA that generate adaptation) seems to peak within _____ after exercise depending on the gene and type of exercise performed.

10. True or False? *(circle one)* Research has shown that training with low muscle glycogen might increase the potential for training adaptations due to triggered reactions such as elevated AMPK activity, but it is unclear if this results in performance improvements.

11. A _____ can reduce or delay symptoms of overreaching, but not completely prevent them.

12. List five potential symptoms of overtraining or overreaching.

a) _____

b) _____

c) _____

d) _____

e) _____

SECTION 4 • **ASSESS YOUR KNOWLEDGE**

1. Endurance training primarily increases protein synthesis related to which of the following components of muscle tissue?

    a. Myofibrils
    b. Mitochondria
    c. Sarcoplasmic reticulum
    d. T-tubules

2. Training adaptations in skeletal muscle are ultimately generated by the cumulative effects of temporary _____ during recovery periods between repeated bouts of exercise.

    a. Increases in lactate and H^+ concentration in muscle tissue
    b. Increases of calcium ion concentration in muscle cytoplasm
    c. Increases in gene transcription onto new proteins
    d. Increases in ATP concentration in muscle tissue

3. Which of the following triggers during exercise can induce the hypertrophy-promoting cytokine known as insulin-like growth factor (IGF)?

    a. Decreased intracellular calcium ion concentration
    b. Decreased AMPK activity
    c. Low reactive oxygen species (ROS) activity
    d. Changes in muscle tension or stretch

4. Changes in protein synthesis (potential adaptation) can begin within hours after exercise but have been shown to last as long as _____.

    a. 8 hours
    b. 15 hours
    c. 24 hours
    d. 48 hours

5. Which of the following compounds that influence molecular signaling (leading to adaptation) cannot function properly with high-dosage antioxidants?

    a. Leucine
    b. ROS
    c. Glycogen
    d. Glutamine

6. The use of medications such as ibuprofen, aspirin, or naproxen for muscle soreness has been shown to potentially suppress protein synthesis by interfering with which of the following processes?

    a. Inflammatory responses that occur after exercise
    b. Calcium flux back into the sarcoplasmic reticulum after exercise
    c. Flushing of H+ out of working tissue after exercise
    d. Mitochondrial energy production

7. Which of the following is NOT a nutrition-related factor that can directly increase the risk for overtraining over time by amplifying the physiological stress response of training?

    a. Glycogen depletion
    b. Excess caloric intake
    c. Inadequate carbohydrate intake
    d. Dehydration

8. Which of the following selections is NOT a symptom directly related to overtraining?

    a. Lack of energy
    b. Insomnia
    c. Increased appetite
    d. Elevated resting heart rate

9. Which of the following is NOT an explicit signal or factor influencing the growth, metabolism, and creation of new muscle proteins?

    a. Heat
    b. Presence of ROS
    c. Nutrient availability
    d. pH in the muscle

10. Which of the following could, in part, initiate increased AMPK activity within muscle cells which in turn can enhance energy metabolism through glucose uptake and fatty acid breakdown?

    a. High ATP concentration within muscle tissue
    b. High calcineurin concentration within muscle tissue
    c. Low AMP concentration within muscle tissue
    d. High ADP concentration within muscle tissue

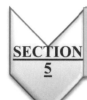

• CHECK YOUR WORK

SPORT NUTRITION CHAPTER 12 ANSWERS

Match the Following Terms

1. D   2. A   3. E   4. B   5. C

Knowledge and Competency Exercises

6. True

7. **a)** Changes occur in muscle stretch or tension, **b)** changes occur in intracellular calcium ion concentrations, **c)** changes occur in the energy charge of a muscle cell, **d)** changes occur in the energy (redox) potential of a muscle cell

8. mRNA

9. 4 to 12 hours

10. True

11. High carbohydrate diet

12. **Possible answers:** Drop in performance, washed-out feeling, tired, drained, lack of energy, mild leg discomfort, general aches and pains in muscles and joints, sleeping problems, insomnia, headaches, decreased immunity, decrease in training capacity or intensity, inability to complete training sessions, moodiness, irritability, and/or depression, loss of enthusiasm for a given sport, decreased appetite, eating problems, increased incidence of injury, reduced maximal lactate and heart rate, elevated resting and sleeping heart rate, no increase in cortisol in response to a stressful bout of exercise

Assess Your Knowledge

1. B   5. B   9. A

2. C   6. A   10. D

3. D   7. B

4. D   8. C

SECTION 1 • LEARNING GOALS

Upon completing this section, along with its corresponding chapter, you should understand the following:

1. The potential effects of body size, body structure, and body composition on sport performance

2. The working definition of body composition

3. The use of body composition assessment among athletic populations

4. Healthy ranges of essential and storage body fat for males and females

5. The use and application of height-weight tables and BMI as indirect measures of disease risk and body composition

6. The use and application of anthropometric measurements to predict body fat

7. The use and application of clinical and field assessments for body composition analysis

• **QUICKFACTS**

OPTIMAL PHYSIQUE FOR SPORT PERFORMANCE

- Body size, structure, and composition are separate yet interrelated aspects of the body that comprise the physique

Body Size	• Refers to the volume, mass, length, and surface area of the body
Body Structure	• Refers to the distribution or arrangement of body parts such as bones, muscle, and fat
Body Composition	• Refers to the amounts of the major constituents of the body, usually including muscle, bone, and fat

- Body composition is the ratio of fat-free mass (FFM) to fat mass (FM)
- Size, structure, and composition can all enhance or negatively affect performance

Body Size	Body Structure
• Specific body size can provide performance advantages depending on the dynamics of a given sport • Examples: jockeys must be small and light, whereas contact sport athletes may find higher body weight advantageous	• Specific variations in body structure provide performance advantages based on demands of a given sport • Example: long wingspan of a basketball center can enhance defensive blocking capability

- There is an inverse relationship between fat mass and performing physical activities that require translocation of body weight vertically or horizontally (jumping or running)
  - Excess fat adds mass to the body without adding capacity to produce force
  - Acceleration is inversely proportional to mass; therefore, excess fat can result in slower changes in velocity and direction
  - Excess fat increases the metabolic cost of physical activities that require total body movement
- **A relatively low percentage of body fat is generally advantageous both mechanically and metabolically; optimal size and structure is dictated by sport-specific dynamics**

Learn More: Sport Nutrition Textbook pg 314

BODY COMPOSITION AND ATHLETICS

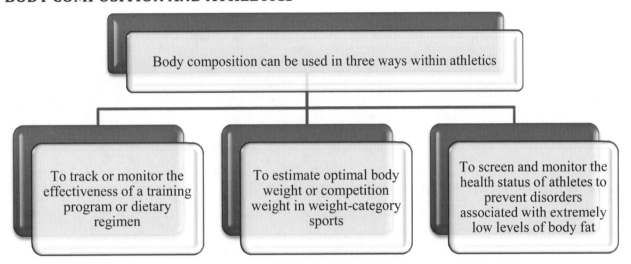

- Table 13.3, pg 316 provides common body fat ranges for both genders in a variety of sports
  - The various ranges reveal that successful athletes have physique characteristics unique to their sport and discipline

Learn More: Sport Nutrition Textbook pgs 315-316

NORMAL RANGES OF BODY FAT
- Body fat consists of essential fat and storage fat

Essential Fat
- Present in nerve tissue, bone marrow, and organs; loss compromises physiological function
- Estimated 3% of body mass for men, 12% for women
- Women have more due to childbearing and hormonal functions

Storage Fat
- Represents an energy reserve that accumulates with excess energy intake

Total Body Fat
- Essential plus storage
- Generally between 12%-15% for young men, 25%-28% for young women

- Differing sports have different requirements in terms of body composition; no accepted standards for percentage of body fat exists for athletes
- Estimates for 'Athletic' classification of body composition – 5%-10% for males, 8%-15% for females; the term athletic refers to sports in which low body fat is an advantage

Learn More: Sport Nutrition Textbook pgs 316-317

Body-Fat Percentages for Males and Females and Their Classification		
Males	Females	Rating
5–10	8–15	Athletic
11–14	16–23	Good
15–20	24–30	Acceptable
21–24	31–36	Overweight
>24	>36	Obese

HEIGHT-WEIGHT TABLES AND BODY MASS INDEX

- **Height-weight tables** – provide a normal range of body weights for any given height but have limited use when applied to the athletic population
    - Do not consider body composition; a heavy, muscular bodybuilder could be considered obese due to 'extra' weight in the form of muscle
- **Body mass index (BMI)** – rough measure used to classify individuals as normal weight, overweight, or obese (still superior to height-weight tables)
    - **BMI = body mass in kilograms ÷ (height in meters)^2**
    - Fails to take into account body composition, so muscular athletes can be interpreted as obese; when used for an individual it should be complemented with other assessments such as waist circumference or skinfold measurements
    - Does provide useful information concerning the risk for various diseases and is used in many epidemiological studies (best used for populations, not individuals)
    - Correlates with the incidence of cardiovascular complications (hypertension and stroke), certain cancers, type 2 diabetes, gallstones, osteoarthritis, and renal disease

Learn More: Sport Nutrition Textbook pgs 317-319

BODY ASSESSMENT TECHNIQUES

- Waist Circumference and Waist-to-Hip Ratio
- Skinfold Measurements
- Hydrostatic Weighing
- Air Displacement Plethysmography
- Bioelectrical Impedance Analysis (BIA)
- Computed Tomography (CT) and Magnetic Resonance Imaging (MRI)
- Dual-Energy X-Ray Absorptiometry (DEXA)

Learn More: Sport Nutrition Textbook pg 317

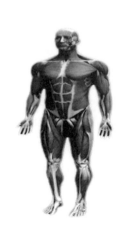

WAIST CIRCUMFERENCE AND WAIST-TO-HIP RATIO

- **Waist-to-hip ratio** – an index of total body fat distribution indicating the level of body fat distributed around the torso
    - o Distribution is evaluated by dividing waist size by hip size; the higher the ratio, the higher the risk for heart disease and other obesity-related disorders
    - o Females – a ratio greater than 0.80 represents a higher risk for disease, a ratio smaller than 0.73 represents a lower risk
    - o Males – a ratio greater than 0.91 represents a higher risk for disease, a ratio smaller than 0.85 represents a lower risk
    - o Example: Person has an 82 cm waist and 78 cm hips: $82 \div 78 = 1.05$ (high risk)
- **Waist circumference** – many studies have found a simple waist circumference measurement to be an optimal indicator of cardiovascular risk factors, body fat distribution, and type 2 diabetes
- These basic measurement are of limited use to most athletic populations

    Learn More: Sport Nutrition Textbook pg 318-319

DENSITOMETRY AND HYDROSTATIC WEIGHING

- **Densitometry** – developed to measure body composition and distinguish the most important bodily components: carbohydrate (usually < 1% of body mass), minerals (~4%), fat (~15%), protein (~20%), and water (~60%)
    - o Each component has a different **density** (mass ÷ volume)
- **Hydrostatic (underwater) weighing** – applies densitometry by using Archimedes' principle of buoyancy (loss of weight in water is equal to the volume of the displaced water); considered the 'Gold Standard' for body composition assessment
    - o Body weight is accurately measured before and after the subject is completely submerged in water; the difference in body weight (equal to weight of displaced water) is used to calculate body fat
    - o Underwater weight must be taken after maximal exhalation (to reduce the buoyancy effect of air in the lungs) and holding the residual breath for 5 to 10 sec
    - o Volume of water displaced must be corrected for the temperature of the water (temperature can change density) and residual lung volume
    - o Food intake should be avoided in the hours before measurement

    Learn More: Sport Nutrition Textbook pgs 319-321

SKINFOLD MEASUREMENTS

- Skinfolds are measured using a special caliper that indicates thickness in mm
- Based on the interrelationships between subcutaneous fat, internal fat, and whole-body density
- A sum of the skinfolds can be used to estimate body fat percentage using the Siri equation
- Various anatomical sites are utilized in differing protocols (3-, 4-, 7- and10-site protocols)
- *Example 3-site protocol:* **males**: chest, abdomen, and thigh; **females**: triceps, suprailiac, and thigh
- When protocol is properly implemented, there is a standard error of only about 3% - 4%
- To ensure accuracy:
    - The skinfold should be taken and the measurement read within 2 seconds to avoid skinfold compression
    - The tester should have considerable experience, and measurements should always be taken by the same person
    - Values that have been established for specific populations (e.g., same gender, same age range, or same ethnicity) must be used

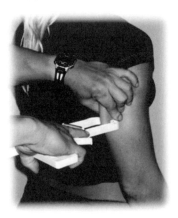

Learn More: Sport Nutrition Textbook pgs 321-324

BIOELECTRICAL IMPEDANCE ANALYSIS (BIA)

- Based on the principle that different tissues provide different resistance to an electrical current
- Electrodes are often placed on the hand and foot and a light, electrical current is ran through the electrodes to measure resistance encountered within the body
    - The lower the resistance, the higher the body water content
    - Adipose tissue has high resistance with low water content; muscle tissue has low resistance with high water content
    - Based on this knowledge, BIA can be used to estimate percentage body fat, percentage lean body mass, and percentage body water

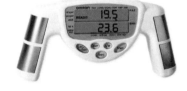

- Optimal assessment protocol:
    - The subject must be lying on a non-conductive surface with the arms not touching the trunk and the legs 20 cm apart
    - Shoes, socks, and metal objects are removed
    - The electrode contact surfaces on the hand and ankle should be cleaned with alcohol
    - Measurement should be performed within 5 minutes of lying down

Learn More: Sport Nutrition Textbook pgs 322, 324-325

CONSIDERATIONS FOR BIOELECTRICAL IMPEDANCE ANALYSIS

- Factors that can negatively affect the validity of the assessment:
    - Differences in skin temperature or sweat on the skin
        - Warmer skin or a wet surface increases conductivity, promoting an underestimation of body fat
    - Hydration status
    - Body position
        - Fluid shifts can affect impedance
- Subjects should be familiar with the following guidelines prior to a BIA assessment:
    - Abstain from alcohol for 8 to 12 hours before the measurement
    - Avoid vigorous exercise for 8 to 12 hours before the measurement
    - Abstain from eating or drinking at least 2 hours before the measurement
    - Void the bowel and bladder before the assessment, if possible
    - Diuretics and menstruation could invalidate the test
- BIA can be a convenient technique, but it requires expertise and control of the testing conditions

Learn More: Sport Nutrition Textbook pgs 324-325

DUAL-ENERGY X-RAY ABSORPTIOMETRY (DEXA)

- Measures body composition based on the principle that compartments of the body with different densities absorb different amounts of low-energy X-rays
- Advantages
    - Very accurate technique that permits estimates of regional composition (arms, legs, trunk, and head) as well as whole-body composition
    - Small changes in composition can be detected
    - Is also the clinical standard for measuring bone mineral density
- Disadvantages
    - Even though it appears to be one of the better methods to measure body composition, testing conditions must be standardized (e.g., hydration status) and commercial DEXA scanners vary, allowing for a source of error
    - Cost prohibitive

Learn More: Sport Nutrition Textbook pg 325

IMAGING TECHNOLOGIES

- **CT** – uses ionizing radiation by an X-ray beam to create images of body segments
- **MRI** – uses electromagnetic radiation to create pictures of body tissues and compartments
- Found to be viable body composition substitutes for more established methods, but calculations derived from scan data is dependent on software, which can produce error

Learn More: Sport Nutrition Textbook pgs 325-326

AIR DISPLACEMENT PLETHYSMOGRAPHY

- Utilizes a small chamber in which air displacement is measured to indicate body volume; commercially marketed as Bod Pod
- Convenient implementation takes only 3-5 min and reproducibility is good
- The subject is first weighed outside of the Bod Pod before sitting inside the 750 L chamber
- Body volume = original volume in chamber – air that has been displaced with subject inside
  - Subject must breathe into an air circuit to assess pulmonary gas volume which is subtracted from measured body volume
- Body density can then be calculated from body mass and volume to indicate composition

Learn More: Sport Nutrition Textbook pg 326

PRACTICAL SUMMARY

- In general, the more complex assessments of body composition are more accurate but unsuitable for conditions outside of the clinical setting
- The gold standards are hydrostatic weighing and DEXA, but the most applicable assessment for athletes in field conditions is the use of skinfold measurements
  - The same person should collect the measurements, and it may be practical to simply examine changes in skinfold total rather than a body fat percentage
- BMI and girth measurements may be useful for unfit individuals and the general population but are not as useful for individual athletes

Learn More: Sport Nutrition Textbook pgs 317-327

SECTION 3 • REVIEW YOUR KNOWLEDGE

Match the Following Terms

1. ___ Body size

2. ___ DEXA

3. ___ Body mass index

4. ___ BIA

5. ___ MRI

6. ___ Body structure

7. ___ Hydrostatic weighing

8. ___ Essential fat

9. ___ Bod Pod

10. ___ Body composition

a. Present in nerve tissue, bone marrow, and organs

b. Arrangement of body parts such as bones or muscle

c. Assesses body composition based on the principle of buoyancy

d. The ratio of fat-free mass to fat mass

e. Skin temperature can affect the validity of this assessment

f. Correlates with the risk for various diseases

g. Measures air displacement to calculate body composition

h. Volume, mass, length, and surface area of the body

i. Is the clinical standard for measuring bone mineral density

j. Can create images of body tissues to assess composition

Knowledge and Competency Exercises

11. List the three aspects of the body that comprise the physique.

a) _____   b) _____   c) _____

12. True or False? *(circle one)* A relatively low percentage of body fat is generally advantageous from a mechanical and metabolic standpoint.

13. Fill in the missing components of the following chart related to body-fat percentage classification.

Males	Females	Rating
5%-10%		Athletic
		Good
	24%-30%	
21%-24%		Overweight
	>36%	Obese

14. List four major components of the body that are differentiated between when implementing densitometry techniques to measure body composition.

a) _____

b) _____

c) _____

d) _____

15. According to the BMI classifications, a value of _____ or higher would signify an individual is obese.

16. List five techniques that directly measure body composition.

a) _____

b) _____

c) _____

d) _____

e) _____

17. True or False? *(circle one)* When skinfold measurements are properly implemented with an experienced tester, there is a standard estimate of error of about 1%-2%.

18. List five guidelines that a subject should be familiar with prior to a BIA assessment.

a) _____

b) _____

c) _____

d) _____

e) _____

19. Fill in the following chart related to techniques to measure body composition.

Method	Description
	Measurement of subcutaneous fat that can give an estimation of FFM and FM
	Measurement of resistance to an electrical current to estimate total-body water, lean body mass, and fat mass
	Use of ionizing radiation by an X-ray beam to create images of body segments

20. True or False? *(circle one)* Even though the gold standards for measuring body composition are hydrostatic weighing and DEXA, the most applicable assessment for athletes in field conditions is skinfold measurement analysis.

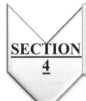

• ASSESS YOUR KNOWLEDGE

1. Which of the following statements regarding the relationship between body composition and sport performance is INCORRECT?

    a.   Excess fat adds mass without improving force production

    b.   Excess fat can result in diminished acceleration capabilities

    c.   Excess fat decreases the metabolic cost of physical activity due to a lower ratio of metabolic tissue in the body

    d.   There is an inverse relationship between fat mass and jumping or running which require forceful translocation of body weight

2. Which of the following is NOT a way in which body composition assessment is constructively used within athletics?

    a.   To assess genetic propensity for elite status in a given sport

    b.   To track the effectiveness of a training program

    c.   To estimate optimal competition weight in weight-category sports

    d.   To monitor the health status of athletes and prevent disorders associated with extremely low levels of body fat

3. Which of the following athletes has the greatest percentage of body fat?

    a.   A ballet dancer with 90 lbs of FFM and 15 lbs of FM

    b.   A football offensive lineman with 200 lbs of FFM and 40 lbs of FM

    c.   A softball player with 125 lbs of FFM and 28 lbs of FM

    d.   A basketball player with 160 lbs of FFM and 16 lbs of FM

4. Which of the following statements related to essential fat is correct?

    a.   Estimated essential fat for men is 8% of body mass

    b.   Men can have a negligible quantity of body fat (<1% of body mass) due to minimal hormonal functions

    c.   Estimated essential fat for women is 4% of body mass

    d.   Women have a greater quantity of essential fat due to childbearing and hormonal functions

5. Which of the following assessments is the least useful for athletes?

    a.   Skinfold measurements

    b.   Hydrostatic weighing

    c.   Bioelectrical impedance analysis

    d.   Waist-to-hip ratio

6. Which of the following assessments could easily classify a very lean, muscular athlete as obese or overweight?

    a. Skinfold measurements
    b. BMI
    c. DEXA scan
    d. Bod Pod

7. Which of the following body composition assessments is known to have the greatest degree of validity (considered a 'Gold Standard')?

    a. Waist circumference measurement
    b. CT scan
    c. Bioelectrical impedance analysis
    d. Hydrostatic weighing

8. Which of the following lists the correct sites to use during a skinfold measurement analysis while implementing a 3-site protocol on a female athlete?

    a. Triceps, suprailiac, and thigh
    b. Biceps, abdominal, and calf
    c. Midaxillary, chest, and thigh
    d. Chest, abdominal, and thigh

9. Hydration status can negatively affect the validity of which of the following body composition assessments?

    a. BMI
    b. Skinfold measurements
    c. CT scan
    d. Bioelectrical impedance analysis

10. Which of the following statements concerning DEXA scanning for assessment of body composition is INCORRECT?

    a. The assessment is based on the principle that compartments of the body with different densities absorb different amounts of low-energy X-rays
    b. The assessment allows for laxity in controlling participant conditions such as hydration status
    c. The assessment permits estimates of regional composition
    d. The assessment allows for small changes in composition to be detected

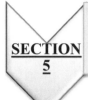

• CHECK YOUR WORK

SPORT NUTRITION CHAPTER 13 ANSWERS

Match the Following Terms

1. H

2. I

3. F

4. E

5. J

6. B

7. C

8. A

9. G

10. D

Knowledge and Competency Exercises

11. a) body size, b) body structure, c) body composition

12. True

13.

Males	Females	Rating
5%-10%	*8%-15%*	Athletic
11%-14%	*16%-23%*	Good
15%-20%	24%-30%	*Acceptable*
21%-24%	*31%-36%*	Overweight
>24%	>36%	Obese

14. a) minerals, b) fat, c) protein, d) water (CHOs are also a component, but found in minimal quantities)

15. 30.0

16. **Possible answers**: Skinfold Measurements, Hydrostatic Weighing, Air Displacement Plethysmography, Bioelectrical Impedance Analysis (BIA), Computed Tomography (CT), Magnetic Resonance Imaging (MRI), and Dual-Energy X-Ray Absorptiometry (DEXA)

17. False

18. a) Abstain from alcohol for 8 to 12 hours before the measurement, b) Avoid vigorous exercise for 8 to 12 hours before the measurement, c) Abstain from eating or drinking at least 2 hours before the measurement, d) Void the bowel and bladder before the assessment if possible, e) Diuretics or menstruation could invalidate the test

19.

Method	Description
Skinfold Measurement Analysis	Measurement of subcutaneous fat that can give an estimation of FFM and FM
Bioelectrical Impedance Analysis	Measurement of resistance to an electrical current to estimate total-body water, lean body mass, and fat mass
Computed Tomography	Use of ionizing radiation by an X-ray beam to create images of body segments

20. True

Assess Your Knowledge

1. C

2. A

3. C

4. D

5. D

6. B

7. D

8. A

9. D

10. B

• LEARNING GOALS

SECTION 1

Upon completing this section, along with its corresponding chapter, you should understand the following:

1. The relationship between genetics and body fat

2. The relationship between adiposity and macronutrient density in the diet

3. The environmental, cultural, and societal factors that can have an effect on adiposity

4. Key terms related to eating behavior including hunger, appetite, satiety, and satiation

5. The mechanisms that regulate eating behaviors and quantity of food intake

6. The effects of exercise on appetite, food intake, metabolism, and weight loss

7. Common dietary, surgical, and pharmaceutical methods for promoting weight loss

8. The pros and cons of common weight loss diets, as well as their usefulness for athletes

9. The metabolic changes that occur when weight loss is attained

10. The concept of weight cycling (yo-yo dieting)

11. Gender differences related to weight loss

12. Strategies to help athletes achieve weight loss without compromising lean mass

13. Common weight loss mistakes made by athletes

14. Factors related to achieving rapid weight loss in weight-category sports

15. Dietary strategies for gaining muscle mass

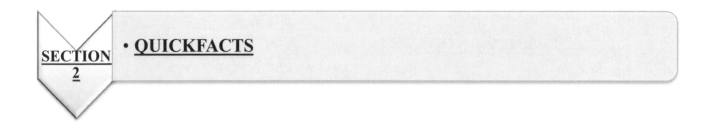

BODY WEIGHT AND COMPOSITION IN DIFFERENT SPORTS REVIEW

- Body size, structure, and composition are separate yet interrelated aspects of the body that comprise the physique
  - o **Body size** – refers to the volume, mass, length, and surface area of the body
  - o **Body structure** – refers to the distribution or arrangement of body parts such as bones, muscle and fat
  - o **Body composition** – refers to the amounts of the major constituents of the body, usually including muscle, bone, and fat
- Size, structure, and composition may enhance or negatively affect performance
- A relatively low percentage of body fat is generally advantageous both mechanically and metabolically; optimal size and structure is dictated by sport-specific dynamics

Learn More: Sport Nutrition Textbook pg 330

GENETICS AND BODY FAT

- 25% to 40% of adiposity is dictated by genetics
- Genetic epidemiology research indicates that genetic factors determine one's susceptibility to gaining or losing body fat
- More than 250 specific genes are believed to potentially influence body fatness

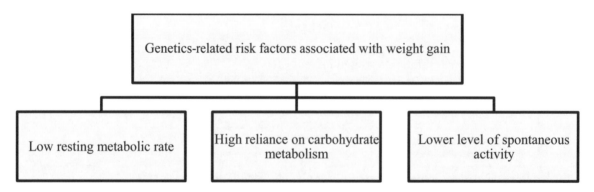

Genetics-related risk factors associated with weight gain

| Low resting metabolic rate | High reliance on carbohydrate metabolism | Lower level of spontaneous activity |

- Relative contribution of genetic vs. environmental factors that affect body fatness is still unclear

Learn More: Sport Nutrition Textbook pg 330

ADIPOSITY AND MACRONUTRIENT INTAKE

- Macronutrient composition in the diet plays an important role in weight management
- CHO or Protein
    - The body immediately increases oxidation rates when excess is ingested
    - Protein is used for synthesizing active tissues/enzymes
    - Both can be deposited as storage fat
- Fat
    - No immediate increase in oxidation rate when excess is ingested
    - Does not generally contribute to active tissue synthesis
    - **Highest propensity to be deposited as storage fat**
- Dietary macronutrient balance can be influenced by the following:
    - Genetics
    - Environmental factors
        - Availability of specific food products
    - Cultural and behavioral differences
        - Many African countries consume a diet containing >70% CHO
        - CHO intake in the US typically equates to 40%-50% of the diet
        - Many sports have a specific eating culture
            - Athletes may be exposed to cafeteria-type foods on a regular basis
            - Alcohol consumption can be part of the sport culture
            - Some sports are characterized by pressure to achieve a low body weight, and striving to reach this goal can result in disordered eating
    - Societal factors
        - Dietary intake differs between socioeconomic classes – lower classes typically have a greater fat intake and lower CHO intake than higher classes

Learn More: Sport Nutrition Textbook pgs 331-332, 334

KEY TERMS RELATED TO EATING BEHAVIORS

Hunger	• Physiological energy need regulated by the brain
Appetite	• Physiological-driven, psychological-based perception of energy need
Satiety	• Refers to the inhibition of eating following a meal; quantified by the measure of time before the next meal • Fiber and protein provide the highest satiety
Satiation	• The sensation of fullness that brings a meal to an end

Learn More: Sport Nutrition Textbook pgs 332-333

REGULATION OF APPETITE AND EATING BEHAVIORS

- Appetite and eating behaviors are centrally regulated by the hypothalamus through the reception and processing of neural, metabolic, and endocrine signals from the body
- Hormone-driven homeostatic mechanisms can influence food intake
  - Hormonal signals from the gastrointestinal (GI) tract
    - Various hormones are released in response to feeding to regulate appetite
      - Examples: cholecystokinin (CCK), glucagon-like peptide-1 (GLP-1), peptide YY (PYY)
  - Hormonal and metabolic signals from specific organs
    - The stomach produces ghrelin to stimulate hunger before eating a meal; after a meal, the hormone returns to baseline concentrations to reduce appetite
    - The liver, pancreas, and intestines also have a subtle influence on food intake
  - Hormonal signals from adipose tissue
    - Insulin and leptin influence feelings of satiety that influence the quantity of food ingested during a given meal
- Neural-driven external factors which exert the <u>strongest</u> influence on the quantity of food intake:
  - Memory
  - Social situations
  - Time of day
  - Stress
  - Taste or smell of food
  - Nutrient content in the meal
  - Exercise or physical activity

Learn More: Sport Nutrition Textbook pgs 332-333

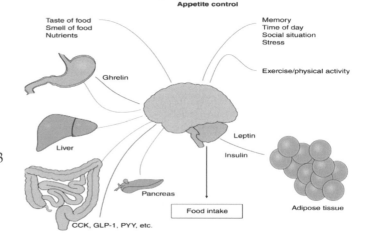

EFFECT OF EXERCISE ON APPETITE AND FOOD INTAKE

- Post-exercise appetite and energy intake depends on many factors
- **Intensity**
  - High-intensity exercise suppresses appetite for a short period after training but does not appear to reduce daily caloric intake long-term
- **Duration**
  - Hunger is only suppressed after long-duration, high-intensity exercise; research suggests 60 min or longer at 70% of VO$_2$max
- **Mode**
  - Treadmill and cycling exercise showed no difference on appetite suppression
  - Anecdotal evidence suggests that swimming increases appetite more than other activities
  - One study compared cycling submerged in cold (20°C) water with cycling in neutral-temperature (33°C) water with increased appetite in the cold conditions

- Exercise-induced reduction in food intake and weight loss
  - Short- to medium-term routine exercise (up to 16 days) is able to produce a negative caloric balance without compensatory responses in food intake
  - Long-term routine exercise (more than 16 days) is likely to cause increased food intake, but the compensation generally only accounts for about 30% of the exercise energy cost
- **Practical Concept**
  - Exercise may be more effective than dieting to produce a negative caloric balance in the short-term (up to 16 days) because compensations in food intake do not usually occur until after a few weeks

Learn More: Sport Nutrition Textbook pgs 332-333

EFFECTS OF EXERCISE ON METABOLISM AND DAILY ENERGY EXPENDITURE

- Exercise increases the resting metabolic rate (RMR) post-exercise, and therefore caloric expenditure
- **Excess Post-exercise Oxygen Consumption (EPOC)**
  - The increase in RMR post-exercise is measured as EPOC
  - Elevation in RMR for a period of time post-exercise is dictated by exercise duration and intensity
  - Longer duration and/or higher intensity (particularly anaerobic exercise) increase the period of time in which EPOC contributes to elevated energy expenditure

Resistance Training	• Can provide an increase in muscle mass and EPOC, increasing daily resting energy expenditure
Aerobic Exercise	• Can change substrate use to facilitate fat loss • Lowers reliance on CHO use and increases capacity to use fat in as little as 4 weeks

Learn More: Sport Nutrition Textbook pgs 333-334

WEIGHT LOSS METHODS

- Many athletes seek to lose body weight, particularly body fat, even when they are not overweight
  - Weight loss can be advantageous for
    - Athletes who need to increase their power-to-weight ratio
      - Beneficial for jumping events
    - Athletes who wish to reduce energy expenditure during prolonged competition
      - Beneficial for runners
  - Weight loss can be detrimental for some athletes
    - It is usually accompanied by a reduction in muscle mass and glycogen stores
    - Can be associated with chronic fatigue and increased risk of injuries
    - Too much emphasis on weight loss can lead to the development of eating disorders

- Weight loss can be attained through the following methods:
  - **Dietary methods**
    - Some proven to be effective, but many provide erroneous assumptions and claims
  - **Exercise**

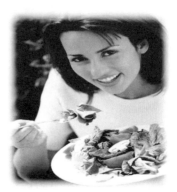

    - When combined with dietary measures, provides the most effective long-term weight loss
  - **Surgical Procedures**
    - Stomach stapling
    - Removal of a section of the small intestine
    - Liposuction
  - **Pharmaceuticals**
    - Stimulants
    - Appetite suppressants
    - Drugs that reduce fat absorption

Learn More: Sport Nutrition Textbook pgs 334-335

WEIGHT LOSS DIETS

- **Very Low-Calorie Diets (VLCDs)**
  - Used as a therapy to achieve rapid weight loss in the obese
  - Liquid meals commonly used contain the recommended daily intake of micronutrients but only 400 kcal/day - 800 kcal/day
    - Meals contain very high protein to reduce muscle wasting, and a relatively small amount of CHO (less than 100 g/day)
  - In the first week, the weight loss is predominantly glycogen and metabolic water even though some fat and protein are also lost
  - After the initial rapid weight loss, weight reduction is mainly from adipose, although loss of body protein continues
    - Increased fat oxidation results in ketosis (formation of ketone bodies) which decreases perception of hunger
  - Side effects can include:

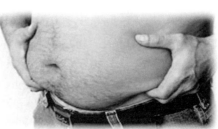

    - Nausea
    - Halitosis (bad breath)
    - Extreme hunger
    - Light-headedness
    - Hypotension
    - Dehydration
    - Electrolyte imbalances
  - **Due to chronic glycogen depletion, loss of muscle mass, and severe reduction in exercise capacity, the diet is unsuitable for athletes**

- **Low-Fat Diets**
  - o Reducing fat intake can be effective for reducing energy intake and promoting weight loss for the following reasons:
    - ▪ Fat energy is dense, providing more than twice the energy per gram than CHO or protein
    - ▪ High-fat foods generally taste good which can promote increased food intake
    - ▪ Fat can be less satiating than protein and most CHOs
    - ▪ Fat is stored efficiently and requires little energy for digestion
    - ▪ Fat intake does not immediately increase fat oxidation
- **Food-Combining Diets**
  - o Based on the philosophy that certain foods should not be combined; most warn against the combining of protein and CHO foods sources
  - o The wrong combinations are stated to cause a "buildup of toxins" with "negative side effects such as weight gain"
  - o It appears that when many of these diets are strictly followed, energy and fat intake are reduced compared to a normal diet – making weight loss success attributed to reduced caloric intake
  - o **Low energy and CHO intake reduces glycogen storage which impairs performance and recovery, making the diet unsuitable for athletes**
- **Low-Carbohydrate Diets**
  - o One of the most well-known low-CHO ketogenic diets is the Atkins diet
  - o Based on the premise that reduced CHO intake will result in increased fat oxidation
  - o Ketone body production increases, suppressing appetite
  - o Low-CHO diets can be effective, but no more than a well-balanced, energy-restricted diet
  - o Not usually recommended due to the relatively high-fat content which can negatively affect the blood lipid profile
  - o **For athletes, these diets are detrimental due to severely reduced glycogen stores and exercise capacity**
- **High-Protein Diets**
  - o Increased protein consumption is a common approach with popular fad diets
  - o A high-protein diet can be effective in supporting weight loss for several reasons
    - ▪ Protein has a greater effect on satiety than CHO or fat
    - ▪ Protein has a greater thermogenic effect than CHO or fat
      - Net metabolism for protein is approximately 3.1 kcal/g – lower than CHO or fat
      - Greater thermogenic effect during digestion enhances fat oxidation
    - ▪ Protein may play a role in maintaining muscle mass during energy restriction, thereby preserving metabolically active tissue
  - o **Overall, evidence suggests that the protein content of a diet can be an important tool in weight management**
- **The Zone Diet**
  - o Proposed by Barry Spears in the book *The Zone: A Dietary Road Map*
  - o Opposes the traditional recommendation of a high-CHO, low-fat diet suitable for athletes
  - o To "enter the zone" the diet should consist of 40% CHO, 30% fat, and 30% protein and be divided into three meals and two snacks per day

- o Due to reduced CHO intake, the diet claims to create an insulin response that provides a favorable insulin-to-glucagon ratio
- o The benefits of this are purported to be:
    - Increased lipolysis
    - Improved regulation of "good" eicosanoids (hormone-like derivates of fatty acids that act as cell-to-cell signaling molecules) and reduction of "bad" eicosanoids
    - Good eicosanoids improve blood flow to working muscle and enhance delivery of O_2 and nutrients
- o Some arguments of the diet are scientifically sound, but the diet has errors, pitfalls, and is based on contradictory data
    - Promised benefits are based on selective data concerning hormonal influences on eicosanoid metabolism while opposing evidence is left out
    - Eicosanoid metabolism is extremely complex and unpredictable, with all previous studies on manipulating synthesis of good forms being unsuccessful
    - The eicosanoid-related benefits purposed are correct in theory but have not been reported in humans; some are theorized assumptions
    - CHO ingestion would have to be lower than 40% to avoid reductions in lipolysis after meals
    - Meals with the 40:30:30 combination are difficult to compose unless the dieter buys the energy bars marketed by Sears
- o **The Zone diet appears to work for some people, most likely due to low energy intake, but the diet is potentially more ergolytic than ergogenic to athletic performance**

PRACTICAL DIET OVERVIEW FOR ATHLETES

- Energy restriction vs. reduced fat intake
    - o When negative caloric balance is achieved, both methods appear equally effective in the long-term
    - o Energy restriction usually results in greater short-term weight loss
- **Conservative caloric restriction via reduced fat intake is the best dietary weight loss method for athletes; high CHO intake can be maintained, resulting in optimal glycogen storage and recovery**
    - o Weight loss should occur slowly and during the off-season

Learn More: Sport Nutrition Textbook pgs 334-337

MANIPULATION OF ENERGY DENSITY
- The energy density of the diet may play an important role in weight maintenance
- Research clearly shows that people tend to eat a similar weight of food regardless of the macronutrient composition
- In a series of studies, Stubbs et al demonstrated that when subjects received a diet that contained either 20%, 40%, or 60% fat, and could eat as they pleased, the weight of the food consumed was nearly identical with each diet
    - o Because of the differences in energy density, the higher-fat diets resulted in greater weight gain

- o The results occurred in both laboratory and free-living conditions
- o Even when the fat content of the subjects' diets was changed but the energy content kept stable, the subjects still consumed the same weight of food

---

EXAMPLE
200g meal (80% CHO, 20% fat) = 1,000kcals x 2 meals/day = **2,000kcals**
200g meal (20% CHO, 80% fat) = 1,600kcals x 2 meals/day = **3,200kcals (+1,200kcals)**

- **Manipulation of energy density is a great tool in weight management or loss**

Learn More: Sport Nutrition Textbook pgs 337-338

CALCIUM AND DAIRY PRODUCTS

- The possible weight-reducing effect of dairy products was first observed by accident during a study investigating the effects of dairy products on hypertension
  - o Subjects who consumed 1,000 mg of calcium/day vs. 400 mg/day lost significant fat
  - o Suggested that dietary calcium can increase fat metabolism by modulating circulating calcitriol (regulates intracellular calcium levels)
  - o Dairy calcium (optimally 1,200 mg/day) appears to be more effective than pill form, suggesting the protein and amino acid content may provide some of the potential weight loss benefit
- The **majority** of current evidence does not support dairy product use for fat loss
  - o Out of 49 randomized trials
    - ▪ 41 showed no effect
    - ▪ 2 demonstrated weight gain
    - ▪ 1 showed a lower rate of weight gain
    - ▪ 5 showed weight loss
- **The specific role of dairy and calcium for weight loss is still unclear**

Learn More: Sport Nutrition Textbook pgs 338-339

USE OF ARTIFICIAL SWEETENERS

- Five artificial sweeteners with intense sweetening power have FDA approval
  - o Acesulfame-K – 200x sweetness of sugar by weight (Nutrinova, FDA-approved 1988)
  - o Aspartame – 160-200x sweetness of sugar by weight (NutraSweet, FDA-approved 1981)
  - o Neotame – 8,000x sweetness of sugar by weight (NutraSweet, FDA-approved 2002)
  - o Saccharin – 300x sweetness of sugar by weight (E954, FDA-approved 1958)
  - o Sucralose – 600x sweetness of sugar by weight (Splenda, FDA-approved 1998)
- Contain minute quantities of energy
- Have the **potential** to reduce energy intake while maintaining palatability of food
- Research suggests that addition to non-energy-yielding products (i.e., diet soda beverages) may actually heighten appetite, but this effect is not seen when ingested with other energy sources

- KEY CONCEPT = Addition to the diet poses no benefit for weight loss or reduced weight gain without energy restriction
- Recent concerns suggest that use of artificial sweeteners may promote additional energy intake and has contributed to obesity, but this has not been substantiated
- **More research is needed to understand the underlying mechanisms, usefulness, and exact effects of artificial sweeteners**

Learn More: Sport Nutrition Textbook pgs 339-340

EXERCISE FOR WEIGHT LOSS

- Dieting alone is ineffective for long-term weight loss, whereas exercise is a favorable way to create a negative energy balance and fat loss
- **Exercise Intensity**
  - Maximal rates of fat use by percentage of calories = 55%-65% of VO$_2$max
  - Greater caloric expenditure and EPOC, but lower fat use at high intensities (>75% of VO$_2$max)
  - Higher intensities better create negative caloric balance
  - Optimal intensity for weight loss is yet to be determined
- **Mode of Exercise**
  - The mode of exercise has been shown to affect maximal rates of fat oxidation
  - Uphill walking and running increased fat oxidation over cycling in multiple studies
  - No long-term studies have been conducted to compare specific modes of exercise and their effectiveness in achieving weight loss
  - **Resistance training appears to be as effective as aerobic exercise for losing fat, but the ultimate factor with either mode is the duration of exercise, which largely determines energy expended**

Learn More: Sport Nutrition Textbook pgs 339-341

METABOLIC CHANGES WITH WEIGHT LOSS

- RMR decreases in response to weight loss, suggesting metabolic changes defend a certain set-point body weight (BW)
- The metabolic response is known as "**food efficiency**" – it serves as an auto-regulatory feedback mechanism to preserve energy and resist additional weight loss
- Makes progressive weight loss increasingly difficult, usually causing a plateau
- In research, BW typically returns to normal in a few weeks after unrestricted eating is again permitted, confirming the set-point BW theory

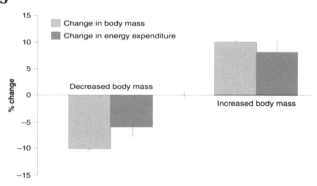

Learn More: Sport Nutrition Textbook pgs 341-342

WEIGHT CYCLING

- Weight cycling (yo-yo dieting effect)
    - o Often the considerable effort applied to achieve weight loss is not followed by the effort required to maintain the new lower body weight
    - o In many cases after weight is lost, it is regained in a relatively short period of time (hence the yo-yo effect reference)
    - o Several prospective studies have shown weight fluctuations are associated with increased mortality independent of the direction of weight change (gain-loss or loss-gain)
    - o Other studies that take limited account of pre-existing disease show little evidence for negative side effects
    - o Overall, it is more dangerous to remain obese than undergo weight cycling

Learn More: Sport Nutrition Textbook pgs 341-342

GENDER DIFFERENCES IN WEIGHT LOSS

- Meta-analyses of studies on weight loss after aerobic exercise showed that weight loss is modestly greater in males
- Gender difference related to weight loss:
    - o Body fat distribution is the primary influence
        - ▪ Women – greater gluteal-femoral storage
        - ▪ Men – greater visceral (abdominal) storage
            - • Fat in the upper body and abdominal regions is more metabolically active and therefore has higher rates of lipolysis in response to exercise
    - o Postprandial (following a meal) fat storage may be higher in subcutaneous adipose tissue in women
- **Due to these physiological variances, women have slightly greater resistance to weight and fat loss**

Learn More: Sport Nutrition Textbook pg 342

WEIGHT LOSS IN ATHLETICS

- Most weight-loss studies have been performed on obese subjects; little evidence has been obtained concerning athletes
- Most athlete weight-loss research focuses on short-term loss for weight-category sports

The first step is to devise clear and practical goals
•It should first be decided if weight loss is really required, and, if so, how much over what period •Body fat should not be reduced below 5% for males or 12% for females •A realistic weight loss time-frame is to lose about 1 lb per week •Rapid (>1lb/week) weight loss will make training difficult and may affect lean mass

- The second step is to establish a clear weight-loss strategy; the following practical guidelines can help athletes achieve realistic weight loss goals
    - Determine a realistic body-weight goal; the help of a sports dietician is likely needed to identify a target weight
    - Do not attempt to lose more than 1 lb per week
    - Do not restrict energy intake by more than 500-750 kcal/day
    - Eat more fruits and vegetables
    - Choose low-fat snacks, and use substitutes for high-fat foods that are currently consumed
    - Limit fatty condiments or add-ons (i.e., sauces, sour cream, salad dressings) or choose low-fat versions
    - Try to structure eating patterns into five or six small meals per day
    - Avoid eating extremely large meals
    - Make sure that CHO intake is high and consume CHO immediately after training
    - A multivitamin and mineral supplement may be useful during energy restriction
    - Measure body weight daily and obtain measurements of body fat regularly (every 2 months) while keeping a record of changes

Learn More: Sport Nutrition Textbook pgs 342-343

COMMON WEIGHT LOSS MISTAKES

- When trying to lose weight, athletes make the following common mistakes:

Trying to lose weight too rapidly	• Results in dehydration and reduced glycogen stores, reducing training capacity • Weight loss without performance loss must occur slowly
Trying to lose weight while in-season	• Commonly results in underperformance; weight loss is best accomplished during the off-season
Skipping breakfast or lunch	• Increases feelings of hunger later in the day • One large evening meal can easily compensate for daytime reduction • Training capacity may diminish due to low liver glycogen stores
Low CHO intake	• When losing body weight there is always the risk of losing muscle mass • This risk can be reduced with relatively large amounts of CHO in the diet which can provide a protein-sparing effect

Learn More: Sport Nutrition Textbook pgs 343-344

MAKING WEIGHT AND RAPID WEIGHT LOSS STRATEGIES

- Making weight is important to athletes in weight-category sports (i.e., wrestling or rowing)
    - o Weigh-ins can take place anywhere from a day before to 30 minutes before competition
    - o In horse racing, jockeys are weighed before and after competition to ensure each horse carries the precise assigned weight – maintaining weight is crucial to competing
    - o Athletes commonly compete at a weight that is 4 - 13 lbs below their normal weight, making rapid weight loss a necessity

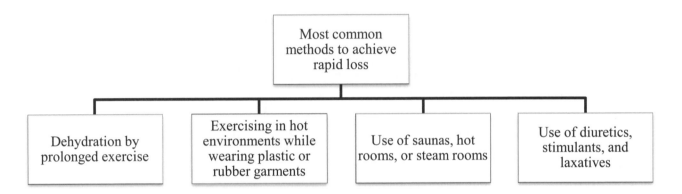

- Rapidly losing weight via these methods can cause the following negative effects (while providing little or no fat loss):
    - o Loss of body water
    - o Reduction in glycogen content
    - o Loss of lean body mass
    - o Reduction in plasma volume
    - o Reduction in central blood volume
    - o Reduction in blood flow to active tissues
    - o Increased core temperature
    - o Increased resting heart rate
    - o Potential for altered hormone status
    - o Impedance of normal growth and development
    - o Impaired psychological state
    - o Potential for impaired academic performance
    - o Impaired immune function

Learn More: Sport Nutrition Textbook pg 344

WEIGHT GAIN IN ATHLETICS

- Concern for athletes in sports where higher body weight and muscle mass is advantageous
    - Examples: hammer throwing, discus throwing, shot put, and weightlifting
- Energy intake must exceed energy expenditure
- To increase lean mass more than fat mass, the athlete must increase CHO intake while limiting additional fat and consume adequate protein
    - Just as the body counteracts a decrease in body weight by decreasing RMR, the RMR increases when energy intake exceeds expenditure
    - Just as large weight losses in a short period of time is unrealistic, so is expecting large weight gains within days
- Realistic weight gains are between 0.4 to 2.0 lb/week, depending on the increase in energy intake
- Synthesis of muscle protein takes a relatively long time (even with excess protein intake) and only occurs in conjunction with resistance training

Learn More: Sport Nutrition Textbook pg 344

SECTION 3 • **REVIEW YOUR KNOWLEDGE**

Match the Following Terms

1. _____ Atkins Diet

a. The sensation of fullness that brings a meal to an end

2. _____ Satiety

b. Hormone released from adipose that regulates satiety

3. _____ Ghrelin

c. Physiological need for energy regulated by the brain

4. _____ Hunger

d. Shown to potentially heighten appetite

5. _____ Satiation

e. Refers to the inhibition of eating following a meal

6. _____ EPOC

f. Appetite-regulating hormone secreted from the stomach

7. _____ Leptin

g. Can significantly reduce glycogen storage and exercise capacity

8. _____ Weight cycling

h. Provides an increase in energy expenditure post-exercise

9. _____ Artificial sweeteners

i. Purposed to modulate eicosanoid function

10. _____ The Zone Diet

j. After weight is lost, it is regained in a short period of time

Knowledge and Competency Exercises

11. List four primary influences related to dietary macronutrient balance.

a) _____   b) _____

c) _____   d) _____

12. True or False? *(circle one)* Fat is the macronutrient with the greatest propensity to be simply deposited as storage fat.

13. List four neural-based external factors that can exert a powerful influence on the quantity of food intake.

a) _____   b) _____

c) _____   d) _____

14. _____ exercise increases the duration of time that EPOC contributes to elevated post-exercise energy expenditure.

15. Describe two ways by which weight loss can be detrimental to athletic performance.

a) _____

b) _____

16. True or False? *(circle one)* Reducing fat intake with conservative caloric restriction is the best fundamental dietary weight loss method for athletes as optimal glycogen storage and recovery can be maintained.

17. List four reasons why simply reducing fat intake can be effective for reducing energy intake and promoting weight loss.

a) _____

b) _____

c) _____

d) _____

18. Very low-calorie diets (VLCDs), food-combining diets, and low-CHO diets may be detrimental to athletic performance due to _____ depletion and impaired _____.

19. List three common methods that weight-category athletes employ to rapidly lose weight.

a) _____   b) _____

c) _____

20. True or False? *(circle one)* Manipulating the energy density of meals can play an important role in weight maintenance as research clearly shows that people tend to eat a lower total quantity of food by weight when the fat content is relatively high.

21. Describe two reasons why females have a slightly greater resistance to weight loss and/or fat loss when compared to males.

a) _____

b) _____

22. Describe four common weight loss mistakes among athletes.

a) _____

b) _____

c) _____

d) _____

23. To "enter the zone" when on the Zone Diet, CHO intake should consist of _____ of daily energy, fat should consist of _____ of daily energy, and protein should consist of _____ of daily energy.

24. List four negative physiological/psychological effects associated with extremely rapid weight loss.

a) _____   b) _____

c) _____   d) _____

25. When attempting to gain weight, an athlete should try to gain between _____ lbs a week with the majority of additional energy intake coming from _____-based food sources.

SECTION 4 • **ASSESS YOUR KNOWLEDGE**

1. Which of the following is a genetic-related risk factor associated with weight gain or obesity?

   a. High level of spontaneous activity
   b. Excess alcohol intake
   c. High reliance on CHO metabolism
   d. High RMR

2. Which of the following is quantified by the measure of time before the next meal?

   a. Hunger
   b. Satiety
   c. Appetite
   d. Satiation

3. Which of the following can exert the most powerful influence on the quantity of food intake during a given meal?

   a. Taste or smell of food
   b. Release of insulin from the pancreas
   c. Release of leptin from adipose tissue
   d. Cytokine signals from the GI tract

4. Which of the following statements related to the effects of exercise on appetite is <u>INCORRECT</u>?

   a. High-intensity exercise suppresses appetite for a short period of time post-exercise
   b. Hunger would be suppressed after a 70-minute aerobic exercise bout performed at 70% of VO_2max
   c. Treadmill exercise has been shown to suppress appetite to a greater degree than cycling when performed at the same intensity
   d. Anecdotal evidence suggests that swimming increases appetite more than most other prolonged activities

5. Which of the following statements concerning very low-calorie diets (VLCDs) is CORRECT?

   a. Daily intake usually ranges from 800kcal-1,500kcal in the form of liquid meals
   b. Meals usually contain very high fat to provide elevated satiety
   c. Diet-induced ketosis related to increased fat oxidation results in heightened appetite
   d. The initial rapid weight loss is predominantly associated with glycogen and metabolic water loss

6. Which of the following diets is purported to reduce the risk of "toxin buildup" from eating the wrong foods?

   a. Low-fat diet
   b. Food-combining diet
   c. Atkins Diet
   d. The Zone Diet

7. Which of the following diets can be effective for losing weight as it can provide relatively high satiety, thermogenic increases in energy expenditure related to digestion, as well as maintenance of muscle mass (even with energy restriction)?

   a. The Zone Diet
   b. Low-fat diet
   c. High-protein diet
   d. Very low-calorie diet

8. _____ decrease(s) in response to weight loss suggesting that metabolic changes attempt to defend a certain set point body weight when an individual is trying to lose weight.

   a. Metabolic hormones
   b. EPOC
   c. Bone mineral density
   d. RMR

9. Which of the following is a proper guideline related to helping an athlete achieve a weight loss goal?

   a. Attempt to lose 2.0-2.5 kg/week for the first few weeks to counteract metabolic compensations related to weight loss
   b. Do not restrict energy intake by more than 150-250 kcal/day
   c. Structure eating patterns into five or six small meals per day
   d. Consume protein-dominant meals immediately after training session

10. Which of the following is <u>NOT</u> an effect of rapid weight loss (seen when athletes lose significant weight just prior to competition)?

   a. Significant reduction in glycogen storage
   b. Significant loss of body fat
   c. Impaired immune function
   d. Reduction in central blood volume

SECTION 5 · CHECK YOUR WORK

SPORT NUTRITION CHAPTER 14 ANSWERS

Match the Following Terms

1. G

2. E

3. F

4. C

5. A

6. H

7. B

8. J

9. D

10. I

Knowledge and Competency Exercises

11. **a)** Genetics, **b)** environmental factors, **c)** cultural differences, **d)** societal factors

12. True

13. **Possible answers:** Memory, social situations, time of day, stress, taste or smell of food, nutrient content in the meal, exercise or physical activity

14. Longer duration and/or higher intensity

15. **a)** It is commonly accompanied by a reduction in muscle mass and glycogen stores, **b)** it can promote chronic fatigue and increased risk of injuries

16. True

17. **Possible answers:** Fat energy is dense, high-fat foods generally taste good which promotes increased food intake, fat can be less satiating than protein and most CHOs, fat is stored efficiently and requires little energy for digestion, and fat intake does not immediately increase fat oxidation

18. Glycogen depletion, exercise capacity

19. **Possible answers:** Dehydration by prolonged exercise, exercising in hot environments while wearing plastic or rubber garments, use of saunas, hot rooms, or steam rooms, use of diuretics, stimulants, and laxatives

20. False

21. **a)** Women store more fat in the gluteal-femoral region which is less metabolically active than upper-body or abdominal adipose tissue, **b)** postprandial fat storage may be higher in subcutaneous adipose tissue in women

22. **a)** Trying to lose weight too rapidly, **b)** trying to lose weight during season, **c)** skipping breakfast or lunch, **d)** taking in too little CHO

23. 40%, 30%, 30%

24. **Possible answers:** Significant loss of body water, reduction in glycogen content, loss of lean body mass, reduction in plasma volume, reduction in central blood volume, reduction in blood flow to active tissues, increased core temperature, increased resting heart rate, altered hormone status, impedance of normal growth and development, impaired psychological state, potential for impaired academic performance, impaired immune function

25. 0.4-2.0, CHO

Assess Your Knowledge

1. C	6. B
2. B	7. C
3. A	8. D
4. C	9. C
5. D	10. B

• LEARNING GOALS

SECTION 1

Upon completing this section, along with its corresponding chapter, you should understand the following:

1. The spectrum of eating behavior

2. The causes, risk factors, negative behaviors, diagnostic criteria, and signs or symptoms associated with clinical eating disorders such as bulimia nervosa or anorexia nervosa

3. The prevalence of eating disorders in athletics

4. The relationship between exercise dependence and eating disorders

5. The negative effects of eating disorders on general health and sports performance

6. Treatment and prevention of eating disorders

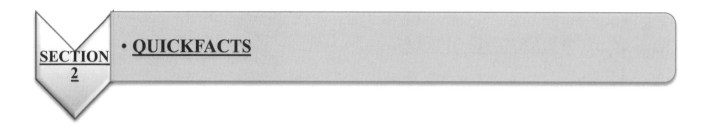

SECTION 2 • **QUICKFACTS**

EATING BEHAVIOR AND DISORDERS

- Eating behavior can be illustrated as a spectrum ranging from excessive **overeating** to **clinical eating disorders**
- Overeating ← healthy (normal) eating → excessive concern over BW → disordered eating → clinical eating disorders

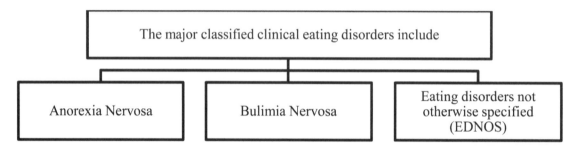

The major classified clinical eating disorders include

Anorexia Nervosa	Bulimia Nervosa	Eating disorders not otherwise specified (EDNOS)

- **Anorexia athletica** – subclinical eating disorder for athletes who show significant symptoms of eating disorders but do not meet the criteria of the *Diagnostic and Statistical Manual of Mental Disorders* for anorexia or bulimia
- Eating disorders are often coupled with psychiatric illnesses (most common among females)

Learn More: Sport Nutrition Textbook pgs 348-349

PRIMARY PROBLEM WITH EATING DISORDERS

- **Low energy availability** – major problem with eating disorders; quantified as dietary energy available for other body functions after exercise training

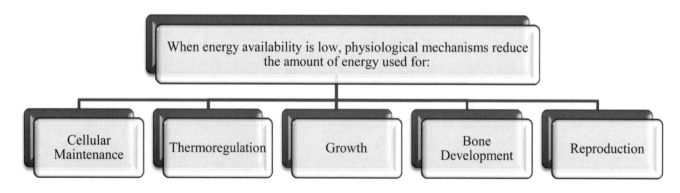

When energy availability is low, physiological mechanisms reduce the amount of energy used for:

Cellular Maintenance	Thermoregulation	Growth	Bone Development	Reproduction

- Compensatory mechanisms tend to restore energy balance and promote survival, but health is significantly impaired
- Athletes reduce energy availability by various means, including:
    o Reducing dietary energy intake
    o Increasing energy expenditure
    o Engaging in abnormal eating behaviors such as fasting, binge eating, or purging
    o Use of drugs such as diet pills, laxatives, and diuretics

Learn More: Sport Nutrition Textbook pgs 348-349

ANOREXIA NERVOSA

- Eating disorder characterized by:
    o Abnormally low food intake
    o Refusal to maintain normal body weight (based on norms for gender, age, and height)
    o A distorted view of body image
    o An intense fear of being overweight and/or gaining weight
    o Having the perception of "feeling fat" when the individual is at least 15% below normal weight for age and height
- **Absence of at least three successive menstrual cycles is a diagnostic criterion**
- Most sufferers do not realize they have a problem and are unlikely to seek treatment
- For the susceptible athlete, it is crucial that the coach, team doctor, sport psychologist, or sports dietitian identify the disorder and persuade the individual to get medical attention

Learn More: Sport Nutrition Textbook pg 349

SYMPTOMS OF ANOREXIA NERVOSA

Physical Symptoms of Anorexia Nervosa or Anorexia Athletica
• Weight loss beyond what is required for optimal sports performance
• Amenorrhea or menstrual dysfunction
• Dehydration
• Excessive fatigue (greater than expected after training or competition)
• Gastrointestinal (GI) problems such as constipation, diarrhea, or distress after meals
• Hyperactivity
• Hypothermia
• Low resting heart rate
• Muscle weakness
• High susceptibility for overuse injuries
• Reduced bone-mineral density and susceptibility to stress fractures
• Frequent infections, skin sores, and poor wound healing
• Low blood hemoglobin and hematocrit, serum albumin and ferritin, glucose, HDL, and estradiol

Psychological Characteristics of Anorexia Nervosa or Anorexia Athletica
• General anxiety • Avoidance of eating and absence from meal situations • Claims of being or feeling fat despite being thin and underweight • Resistance to recommendations for weight gain • Unusual weighing behaviors (e.g., excessive weighing, avoidance of weighing, negative reaction to being weighed, refusal to be weighed) • Excessive training beyond that required for a particular sport • Exercising while injured or when prohibited by coaching and medical staff • Obsessed about body image • Compulsive behaviors regarding eating and physical activity • Restlessness and inability to relax • Social withdrawal, irritability, and/or depression • Tiredness and insomnia

Learn More: Sport Nutrition Textbook pg 349

BULIMIA NERVOSA

- Eating disorder behaviors
  - o Individual engages in repeat cycles of **binge eating** (consumption of large amounts of usually energy-dense foods)
  - o Followed soon after by **purging** of the stomach contents (vomiting) before many of the nutrients can be absorbed (not characteristic of all bulimics)
  - o The person often eats food in secrecy and commonly disappears from view shortly after a meal to purge the contents

Other compensatory behaviors include:	Prolonged fasting	Excessive exercise	Use of laxatives and diuretics

- Many bulimic athletes maintain a normal body weight; the athlete's support team must be able to identify physical symptoms and psychological characteristics
  - o Bulimic athletes do not usually disclose information about their abnormal behavior until they perceive the habit is negatively affecting sports performance
  - o Many bulimics go undetected

Learn More: Sport Nutrition Textbook pg 349

SYMPTOMS OF BULIMIA NERVOSA

Physical Symptoms of Bulimia Nervosa
•Calluses, sores, or abrasions on fingers or back of hand used to induce vomiting •Dehydration •Dental or gum problems •Edema, complaints of bloating, or a combination of the two •Serum electrolyte abnormalities •GI problems •Low weight despite apparent intake of large amounts of food •Frequent and often extreme weight fluctuations •Muscle cramps and/or muscle weakness •Swollen parotid salivary glands •Menstrual irregularities in females

Psychological Characteristics Associated with Bulimia Nervosa
•Binge eating •Secretive eating and agitation when binging is interrupted •Disappearing after eating meals •Evidence of vomiting unrelated to illness •Dieting •Excessive exercise beyond that required for the athlete's sport •Depression •Self-critical, especially concerning body image, body weight, and sports performance •Substance abuse •Use of laxatives, diuretics, or both that are unsanctioned by medical or coaching support staff

Learn More: Sport Nutrition Textbook pgs 349-350

EATING DISORDER NOT OTHERWISE SPECIFIED (EDNOS)

- Used to classify individuals who do not meet all the criteria for anorexia or bulimia nervosa
- Individual may meet all the criteria for anorexia nervosa **except** she has regular menses
- Individual may meet all the criteria for bulimia nervosa **except** he or she binges and purges less than 2x/week
- Sufferers will present with many symptoms that have the potential to diminish performance

Learn More: Sport Nutrition Textbook pg 350

PREVALENCE OF EATING DISORDERS

- Current data on the prevalence of eating disorders is limited as minimal research has applied strict classification criteria (such as used in the *Diagnostic and Statistical Manual of Mental Disorders*) to athletes or non-athletes

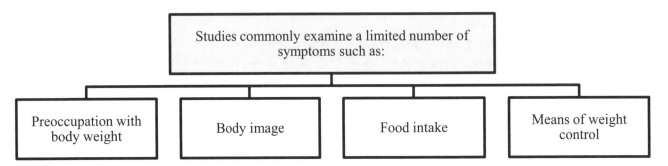

- Research does indicate
  - A substantially greater incidence among athletes when compared with non-athletes and females when compared with males
  - Bulimia nervosa and subclinical eating disorders are more prevalent among female athletes when compared to non-athletes
  - Prevalence of anorexia nervosa is identical for female athletes and non-athletes
- Eating disorders are **most** common among females who compete in endurance, weight-category, and aesthetic sports
  - Related to importance of leanness to succeed or the perceived advantage of competing in a lower weight-category
  - Less common among females who compete in team, power, and technical sports

Learn More: Sport Nutrition Textbook pg 350

CAUSES AND RISK FACTORS FOR EATING DISORDERS

- The precise causes of eating disorders are not known, but they probably progress from an initial desire or requirement to lose weight that develops into a pathological fear of gaining weight
  - Highly motivated and hard driven young females are at the highest risk
- Factors that increase the risk for eating disorders:
  - **Gender**
    - Most significant risk factor
    - Evidence shows that females may have a 10x greater risk than males, but incidence among males is on the rise
  - **Lifestyle**
    - Competing in a sport in which being thin or maintaining a low body weight is considered essential to success
  - **Dieting**
    - One study showed that girls who engaged in a severe diet were 18x more likely to be diagnosed with a clinical eating disorder 6 months later

- o **Personality traits**
  - Most people with eating disorders are reported to have low self-esteem and to be excessively self-critical about body image
  - Many have "control issues" where they feel food/exercise is one of the only controllable factors in their lives
  - Bulimia sufferers consistently show high levels of impulsivity and their addictiveness scores resemble those of drug addicts
  - Some traits that encourage good sports performance can also lead to an unnatural preoccupation with body image and fatness
    - Perfectionism
    - Dedication
    - Willingness to work excessively hard
    - Ability to withstand significant discomfort

Learn More: Sport Nutrition Textbook pgs 351-352

EXERCISE DEPENDENCE AND EATING DISORDERS

- Excessive exercise is widely reported to coexist with eating disorders, particularly among those who practice dietary restraint
  - o Example: **Body dysmorphic disorder** - condition where males are not happy with their bodies and are prepared to engage in excessive exercise, supplement use, and drug abuse to increase muscle, look leaner, and attain a lean muscular midsection
- Over-activity among those with eating disorders appears in multiple ways
  - o Deliberate exercise to increase energy expenditure and promote fat loss
    - In this case, exercise is considered a secondary symptom of the disorder
  - o Involuntary and persistent restlessness that often causes sleep disturbances
    - May be a central feature of the disorder
- **High levels of exercise/activity seems to play an important role in the perpetuation of an eating disorder**

Learn More: Sport Nutrition Textbook pg 352

EFFECTS OF EATING DISORDERS ON SPORT PERFORMANCE

- The effects of an eating disorder on sports performance are determined by the length and severity of the disorder as well as the nature of the sport (i.e., predominant requirement being power, strength, endurance, or motor skills)
- Athletes with eating disorders may:
  - o Have diminished liver and muscle glycogen stores
  - o Be consistently dehydrated
    - Affects all components of performance (even motor skills and coordination)
    - Impairs thermoregulation during exercise
  - o Become anemic (when blood hemoglobin concentration falls below normal)

o Exhibit electrolyte imbalances
o Lose significant muscle, therefore impairing strength and power
- **Both short-term, high-intensity and endurance exercise performance are negatively affected**

Learn More: Sport Nutrition Textbook pgs 352-353

EFFECTS OF EATING DISORDERS ON HEALTH

- Eating disorders can cause many health problems for athletes due to:
  o Reduced energy availability
  o Micronutrient deficiencies
    - For female athletes in particular, inadequate intake of calcium, iron, and B vitamins is often a serious concern
- Eating disorders can affect numerous physiological functions
- **Psychological mood state**
  o Depression is a common symptom
  o Increased fatigue, anxiety, anger, and irritability are associated with low energy and CHO intake
- **Growth and maturation**
  o The onset of puberty may be delayed in child athletes
  o Severely stunted growth can occur in adolescent athletes
  o Poor bone development can increase the susceptibility of fractures later in life
- **Reproductive function**
  o Female reproductive function is affected by negative energy balance, psychological stress, and low body-fat content
  o The ovarian production of sex the steroid hormones estrogen and progesterone drops to extremely low levels during prolonged energy deficits
  o Lack of ovarian hormone production can cause athletic amenorrhea or infertility
- **Bone health**
  o Because ovarian steroid hormones facilitate calcium uptake into bone and inhibit bone resorption, amenorrhea is associated with an increased risk for osteoporosis
  o The weight-bearing effects of athletic training that usually protect against osteoporosis cannot adequately offset the effects of low ovarian hormones
  o Dietary inadequacy and disruption of the normal menstrual cycle during the pubertal growth spurt will have the <u>most severe</u> impact on bone formation and peak bone mass
  o Development of osteoporosis is accelerated by inadequate intake of vitamin D or calcium commonly seen with eating disorders
    - Calcium should be increased to 120% of the RDA in women with amenorrhea
- **Mortality**
  o Specific death rates from eating disorders among athletes are not known
  o Among patients with anorexia nervosa in the general population, mortality is reported to range from <1% - 18%
  o With anorexics, death is usually caused by excessive fluid/electrolyte disturbance (increases risk for cardiac arrest) or suicide

- o Data on mortality in bulimia nervosa is not available, but deaths usually occur as a complication of vomiting behavior or suicide
- Amenorrhea, disordered eating, and osteoporosis are collectively known as the **female athlete triad syndrome**
  - o Any female athlete is at risk, but those who participate in sports where low body fat is advantageous are at highest risk

Learn More: Sport Nutrition Textbook pgs 353-357

TREATMENT AND PREVENTION OF EATING DISORDERS

- General prevention and treatment considerations:
  - o Early diagnosis is vital as disorders become more difficult to treat over time
  - o Most effective means of preventing/treating eating disorders among athletes is **education**
    - ▪ Risks, negative effects on health/performance, balanced meal planning, and normal eating patterns should be addressed
  - o Eating disorders may persist even after education/counseling as they often are complex examples of psychological dysfunction
  - o Exercise dependence and depression are common side issues
  - o Coaches must understand their influence on an athlete's eating and weight-control behaviors

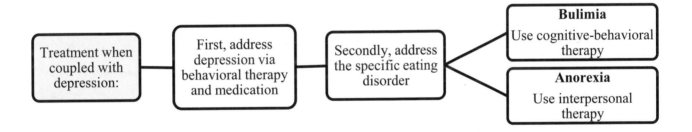

- After diagnosis and initial treatment:
  - o Athletes should maintain a BW no less than 90% of "ideal" health-related BW
  - o Those who have been amenorrheic for more than 6 months should:
    - ▪ Have their bone-mineral density measured
    - ▪ Be considered for hormone replacement therapy
  - o Refer to a dietician for nutrition counseling and to estimate energy availability

Learn More: Sport Nutrition Textbook pg 357

• **REVIEW YOUR KNOWLEDGE**

Match the Following Terms

1. _____ Anorexia nervosa
a. Characterized by binge eating; often followed by self-induced vomiting

2. _____ Binge eating
b. Includes osteoporosis, amenorrhea, and disordered eating

3. _____ Body dysmorphic disorder
c. Quantified as energy used for bodily functions after exercise

4. _____ Bulimia nervosa
d. Refers to the emptying of stomach contents

5. _____ Purging
e. When diminished, can increase the risk for osteoporosis

6. _____ Energy availability
f. Consumption of large amounts of food

7. _____ Female triad syndrome
g. Characterized by extremely low food intake

8. _____ Estradiol
h. Eating/psychological disorder more common among males

Knowledge and Competency Exercises

11. What are the three classified clinical eating disorders?

a) _____   b) _____   c) _____

12. Fill in the blanks of the eating behavior spectrum.

_____ ← healthy (normal) eating → _____ → disordered eating → _____

13. List three physiological functions that are negatively affected with low energy availability.

a) _____   b) _____   c) _____

14. True or False? *(circle one)* Anorexia nervosa is characterized by abnormally low food intake, a distorted body image, and an intense fear of gaining weight.

15. List four physical symptoms associated with anorexia nervosa.

a) _____   b) _____

c) _____   d) _____

16. True or False? *(circle one)* Many bulimic athletes actually maintain a normal body weight.

17. List four psychological symptoms associated with bulimia nervosa.

a) _____   b) _____

c) _____   d) _____

18. An individual diagnosed with an EDNOS may meet all the criteria for bulimia nervosa except he or she _____; or for anorexia nervosa except she _____.

19. True or False? *(circle one)* Eating disorders are <u>most</u> common among power and technical skill sports.

20. Describe two ways in which eating disorders can negatively affect an athlete's performance.

a) _____

b) _____

21. _____ and _____ are two minerals of serious concern (as it relates to deficiency) among female athletes with an eating disorder.

22. Athletes who have been amenorrheic for more than 6 months should have their _____ measured and be considered for _____ therapy.

1. Which of the following is a diagnostic criterion for anorexia nervosa?

    a.   A degree of restlessness that results insomnia
    b.   Low HDL cholesterol
    c.   The absence of three consecutive menstrual cycles
    d.   Consistently eats small meals throughout the day

2. Which of the following is a psychological characteristic associated with anorexia nervosa?

    a.   Binge eating
    b.   Unusual weighing behaviors
    c.   Evidence of vomiting unrelated to illness
    d.   Dehydration

3. Which of the following describes why an individual with bulimia nervosa is at a relatively high risk for nutrient deficiencies?

    a.   Bulimia nervosa sufferers generally refuse to eat food for 3-4 hours after a training session
    b.   Bulimia nervosa sufferers generally self-dehydrate due to an inherent fear of fluid-induced bloating
    c.   Bulimia nervosa sufferers generally engage in repeat cycles of binge eating
    d.   Bulimia nervosa sufferers generally purge the contents of the stomach before many nutrients can be absorbed

4. Which of the following is a physical symptom <u>most</u> specific to an individual who suffers from bulimia nervosa?

    a.   Calluses, sores or abrasions on the back of the hands
    b.   Hypothermia
    c.   Depression
    d.   Infertility

5. Which of the following does <u>NOT</u> reflect research findings examining the prevalence of eating disorders?

    a.   Eating disorders are more prevalent among athletes when compared to the general population
    b.   Eating disorders are more prevalent among females when compared to males
    c.   Prevalence of anorexia nervosa is more common among male non-athletes when compared to male athletes
    d.   Prevalence of bulimia nervosa is more common among female athletes when compared to female non-athletes

6. Which of the following is considered the most significant risk factor for being diagnosed with an eating disorder?

    a. Lifestyle
    b. Dieting
    c. Personality traits
    d. Gender

7. Eating disorders can reduce athletic performance <u>mainly</u> due to _____.

    a. Reduced protein synthesis
    b. Low energy availability
    c. Lack of motivation
    d. Reduced anabolic hormone activity

8. Which of the following describes a major reason why the risk for osteoporosis is elevated among individuals who suffer from an eating disorder?

    a. The ovarian production of sex steroid hormones estrogen and progesterone drops to extremely low levels during prolonged energy deficits
    b. The high levels of associated psychological stress modify circulating leptin actions
    c. Gonadotropic hormone production is increased in response to energy deficit
    d. Testosterone production is increased, promoting calcium resorption in bone among females

9. Which of the following is a primary cause of death among anorexics?

    a. CNS failure from glycogen depletion
    b. Complications associated with vomiting behavior
    c. Cardiac arrest due to excessive fluid/electrolyte disturbance
    d. Fractures

10. Which of the following statements concerning the body dysmorphic disorder is <u>INCORRECT</u>?

    a. Sufferers are willing to engage in drug abuse to attain a leaner appearance
    b. Sufferers commonly engage in excessive exercise and supplement use to increase muscle
    c. Sufferers are continually unhappy with their physique
    d. The disorder is most common among females

• CHECK YOUR WORK

SPORT NUTRITION CHAPTER 15 ANSWERS

Match the Following Terms

1. G

2. F

3. H

4. A

5. D

6. C

7. B

8. E

Knowledge and Competency Exercises

11. **a)** Anorexia nervosa, **b)** bulimia nervosa, **c)** EDNOS

12. *Overeating* ← healthy (normal) eating → *excessive concern over BW* → disordered eating → *clinical eating disorders*

13. **Possible answers:** Cellular maintenance, thermoregulation, growth, bone development, reproduction

14. True

15. **Possible answers:** Weight loss beyond what is required for optimal sports performance, amenorrhea or menstrual dysfunction, dehydration, excessive fatigue (greater than expected after training or competition), gastrointestinal (GI) problems such as constipation, diarrhea, or distress after meals, hyperactivity, hypothermia, low resting heart rate, muscle weakness, high susceptibility for overuse injuries, reduced bone-mineral density

and susceptibility to stress fractures, frequent infections, skin sores, and poor wound healing, low blood hemoglobin and hematocrit, as well as low serum albumin, serum ferritin, glucose, HDL cholesterol, and estradiol levels

16. True

17. **Possible answers:** Binge eating, secretive eating and agitation when binging is interrupted, disappearing after eating meals, evidence of vomiting unrelated to illness, dieting, excessive exercise beyond that required for the athlete's sport, depression, self-criticism (especially in regards to body image, body weight, and a decline in sports performance), substance abuse, use of laxatives, diuretics, or both that are unsanctioned by medical or coaching support staff

18. Binges and purges less then 2x/week, has regular menses

19. False

20. **Possible answers:** The athlete may have diminished liver and muscle glycogen stores, the athlete may be consistently dehydrated, the athlete can become anemic, the athlete may exhibit electrolyte imbalances, the athlete can lose significant muscle, therefore impairing strength and power

21. Calcium, iron

22. bone-mineral density, hormone replacement

Assess Your Knowledge

1. C

2. B

3. D

4. A

5. C

6. D

7. B

8. A

9. C

10. D

• LEARNING GOALS

SECTION 1

Upon completing this section, along with its corresponding chapter, you should understand the following:

1. The functions of the immune system

2. The differences between the innate and adaptive components of the immune system

3. The actions that occur during an immune response

4. The factors that lead to immunodepression among competitive athletes

5. The acute and chronic effects of exercise on immune function

6. Practical strategies that minimize the risk of infection directly after a training session and throughout the competitive season

7. Nutritional influences on immune function among competitive athletes

8. The effects of carbohydrate, fat, protein, alcohol, caffeine, vitamins, antioxidants, and minerals on immune function

9. The potential benefits of dietary immunostimulants and other supplements on immune function

SECTION 2 • **QUICKFACTS**

FUNCTIONS AND COMPONENTS OF THE IMMUNE SYSTEM

- The immune system is involved in:
  - Tissue recovery and repair after injury
  - Protection of the body against potentially damaging (pathogenic) organisms such as bacteria, viruses, and fungi
- The immune system recognizes, attacks, and destroys all foreign materials
- The immune system has two broad "subsystems" with specific functions
- **Innate immunity**
  - Activated when an infectious agent attempts to enter the body (first line of defense)
  - Comprised of three general mechanisms to prevent microorganism entry into the body
    - Physical or structural barriers such as skin or mucosal secretions
    - Chemical barriers such as the pH of bodily fluids
    - Phagocytic cells – consume microorganisms
- **Adaptive immunity**
  - Activated with failure of innate immunity by consequential infection
  - Aids infection recovery via lymphocyte actions that:
    - Recognize the foreign/infectious molecules (**antigens**) to attack
    - Produce an immunological "memory" response that enables the immune system to mount an augmented response when the body is re-infected by the same pathogen
- **Cellular** and **soluble** elements function in both components of the immune system

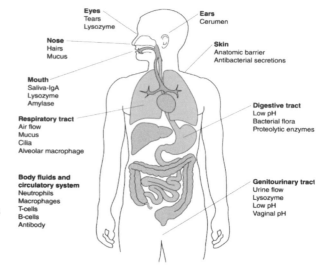

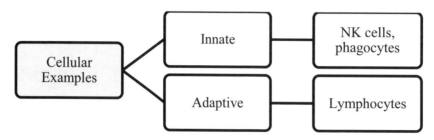

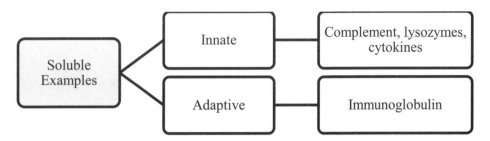

Learn More: Sport Nutrition Textbook pgs 362-364

THE IMMUNE RESPONSE

- An infectious agent in the body first initiates an **inflammatory response** which:
    - Increases local blood flow to the infected area
    - Increases permeability of local capillaries
    - Allows entry of white blood cells (WBCs), or leukocytes, and plasma proteins into the infected tissue
- Immune responses vary based on the type of infectious agent (parasitic, bacterial, fungal, or viral)
- Macrophages are key players
    - They first ingest invading microorganisms to metabolize proteins on its surface
    - They then activate lymphocytes and antibodies specifically designed to eradicate the infectious agent
- Innate defense mechanisms such as NK cells and neutrophils are activated
- Cytokine release triggers numerous immune cells and inflammatory mediators
- B-cell lymphocyte stimulation results in the creation of antibody-secreting cells which are essential to antigen recognition and immunological memory responses

Learn More: Sport Nutrition Textbook pgs 364-370

EXERCISE AND THE IMMUNE SYSTEM

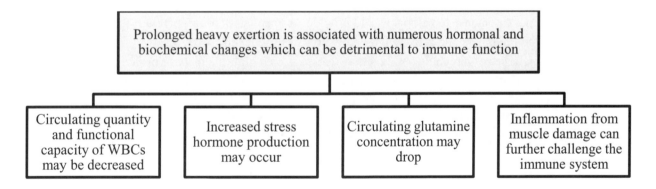

- Performance-impairing **immunodepression** (suppressed immune function) and the increased incidence of infection among athletes is multifactorial
- **Physical**
  - Heavy endurance training increases the incidence of upper respiratory tract infections (URTIs)
  - Sore throats and flu-like symptoms are more common among athletes
- **Environmental**
  - Training and competitive surroundings may increase the athlete's exposure to pathogens such as airborne bacteria or viruses while providing optimal conditions for transmission (exacerbated by higher rate and depth of breathing)
  - Prolonged training in the heat can increase gut permeability which can allow gut bacteria endotoxins to enter circulation
- **Psychological**
  - The psychological demands of training and pressure to succeed (anxiety) can affect stress hormone dynamics
- **Nutritional**
  - Deficiencies and/or nutrition excess can impair immune function and increase the risk for infections

Learn More: Sport Nutrition Textbook pgs 362, 371-372

ACUTE EFFECTS OF EXERCISE ON IMMUNE FUNCTION

- An acute bout of exercise results in responses that are similar, in many respects, to those induced by infection, including:
  - Increased circulating WBCs; magnitude is related to the intensity and duration
  - Increased release of various substances that influence WBC functions, such as C-reactive protein and cytokines
  - Hormone changes including increases in the plasma concentration of adrenaline, cortisol, growth hormone, and prolactin, all of which have immunomodulatory effects
  - Temporary increase in NK cell activity
- The following changes occur during the early recovery period after exercise which appear to weaken the potential immune response to pathogens and provide an open window for infection for the athlete:
  - NK cell numbers and activity fall below pre-exercise levels
  - The number of circulating WBCs may decrease with high-intensity or prolonged exercise
  - Plasma glutamine falls by about 20% and may remain depressed for many hours
  - Temporary reductions in many aspects of innate immunity function occur

Learn More: Sport Nutrition Textbook pgs 372-373

MINIMIZING RISK FOR INFECTION OR ILLNESS AFTER EXERCISE

Athletes are encouraged to adopt the following practices to minimize risk of infection after a training session
• Avoid contact with people who have symptoms of infection • Minimize contact with school-age children and large crowds • Wash hands regularly, particularly after touching surfaces frequently handled by others (i.e., doorknobs, handrails, etc) • Avoid hand-to-eye and hand-to-mouth contact to prevent transferring microbes to sensitive mucosal tissues • Maintain good oral hygiene • Avoid getting a dry mouth during competition and at rest by drinking at regular intervals and maintaining hydration status • Never share drink bottles or cutlery • Use properly treated water for consumption and swimming • Avoid shared saunas, showers, and whirlpool tubs • Remain aware that good personal hygiene and thoughtfulness are the best defenses against respiratory infections

Learn More: Sport Nutrition Textbook pg 373

CHRONIC EFFECTS OF EXERCISE TRAINING ON IMMUNE FUNCTION

- Exercise training can promote long-lasting immunodepressive effects
    - Circulating WBC counts are generally lower in athletes at rest when compared with sedentary individuals
        - Can occur from expansion of blood volume associated with training or diminished release from bone marrow
    - Neutrophil reserves in bone marrow can become depleted over a period of long-term, heavy training
    - The blood population of immune cells seems to be less mature among athletes
    - Phagocytic (digestion of microbes) activity of blood neutrophils has been reported to be markedly lower in well-trained cyclists when compared with control subjects
- Several causes/mechanisms of the reduction in immune function associated with heavy training are possible:
    - The cumulative effects of repeated bouts of intense exercise, with the subsequent elevation of stress hormones (particularly glucocorticoids) can cause immunodepression without sufficient time for system recovery
    - Plasma glutamine levels can become chronically depressed after repeated bouts of prolonged strenuous training
    - Repeated muscle damage can contribute to chronically decreased innate immunity function

Learn More: Sport Nutrition Textbook pgs 373-374

NUTRITIONAL INFLUENCES ON IMMUNE FUNCTION IN ATHLETES

- Nutrient availability can significantly affect the immune system as many nutrients are involved in energy metabolism and protein synthesis
    - Most immune responses involve cell replication and production of proteins with specific functions (e.g., cytokines, antibodies, and acute phase proteins)
- Immune system functions that may be compromised
    - Antibody production
    - Inter-cellular immunity
    - Capacity of phagocytes to kill bacteria
    - Complement formation – found in serum, consisting of 20 or more proteins that stimulate neutralization of infected cells
    - Lymphocyte creation
- A nutritional deficiency is either classified as:
    - **Having a direct effect on immune function**
        - When the nutritional factor has primary activity within the **lymphoid system** (part of the immune system comprised of a network of conduits called lymphatic vessels that carry a clear fluid called lymph, and the structures that are dedicated to the circulation and production of lymphocytes, such as the spleen and tonsils)
    - **Having an indirect effect on immune function**
        - When the nutritional factor affects all cells or an organ system that functions as an immune regulator
    - Example – Carbohydrate (CHO) availability
        - **Directly** effects WBC functions
        - **Indirectly** affects the lymphoid system through its influence on circulating levels of catecholamines and cortisol

```
┌─────────────────────────────────────────────────────────────────────┐
│       The effect of a nutrient deficiency on the immune system depends on       │
└─────────────────────────────────────────────────────────────────────┘
        ┌───────────────────────────────┴───────────────────────────────┐
┌───────────────────────────────────┐          ┌───────────────────────────────────┐
│ The duration and severity of the  │          │ The athlete's nutritional status  │
│            deficiency              │          │           as a whole              │
└───────────────────────────────────┘          └───────────────────────────────────┘
```

- Additional considerations:
    - The availability of one nutrient may enhance or impair the action of another
    - Nutrient deficiencies commonly occur together, making nutrient-to-nutrient interactions on immune function important to understand
    - Excess intake of specific nutrients such as iron or zinc can have detrimental effects on immune function

Learn More: Sport Nutrition Textbook pgs 374-375

CARBOHYDRATE AND IMMUNE FUNCTION

- Adequate CHO availability is necessary for maintenance of heavy training schedules and successful athletic performance
    - Athletes should consume enough CHO to cover 60% of their energy cost
    - Optimal daily intake is 8-10 g/kg of BW for athletes who train for >2 hours/day
    - Adequate glucose is necessary to properly fuel cells of the immune system which have extremely high metabolic rates

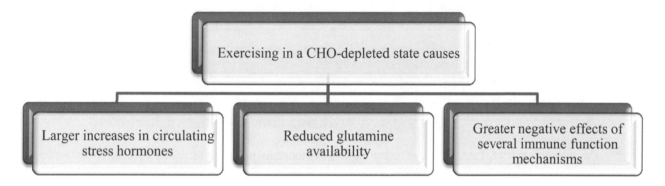

- Consuming CHO (but not glutamine) during exercise helps reduce stress hormones and appears to limit the degree of exercise-induced immunodepression

Learn More: Sport Nutrition Textbook pgs 375-378

FAT AND IMMUNE FUNCTION

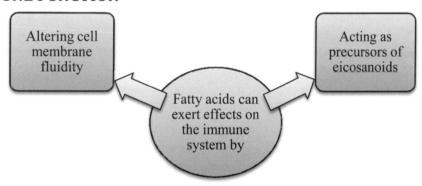

- Little is clearly known about the contribution of FAs to the regulation of exercise-induced alteration of immune function
- Omega-3 and Omega-6 polyunsaturated fatty acids (PUFAs) have immunomodulatory functions
    - Shown to improve the conditions of patients suffering from diseases characterized by an overactive immune system such as rheumatoid arthritis
    - Excessive intake may increase the exercise-induced suppression of cytokine and lymphocyte production due to anti-inflammatory dynamics

Learn More: Sport Nutrition Textbook pgs 378-379

PROTEIN AND IMMUNE FUNCTION

- Athlete needs are about 2x that of sedentary individuals
- Daily intake of <1.6g/kg of BW is likely to be associated with a negative nitrogen balance in athletes with intense training regimens
- Glutamine (abundant amino acid) is utilized at extremely high rates by WBCs
- Inadequate protein intake can significantly impair immunity as clearly seen during protein-energy malnutrition (PEM)
  - Detrimental effects on T-cell lymphocyte functions that protect from infection
  - Widespread atrophy of lymphoid tissue
  - Impaired phagocytic immune cell function
  - Decreased cytokine production
  - Reduced complement formation
- **Athletes are unlikely to encounter extreme protein malnutrition unless on a severely restricted diet, but immunity impairment is observed even with moderate-protein deficiency**

Learn More: Sport Nutrition Textbook pgs 379-380

EFFECTS OF ALCOHOL AND CAFFEINE ON IMMUNE FUNCTION

- **Alcohol**
  - High consumption can directly suppress a wide range of immune responses
  - Abuse is associated with an increased number of infectious diseases
  - Moderate intake appears beneficial for immune function compared with abstinence
  - The ethanol in alcoholic beverages may have detrimental effects, while the polyphenol compounds may have anti-inflammatory effects
  - **Evidence suggests that consumption of light to moderate amounts of polyphenol-rich alcoholic beverages such as wine and beer could have health benefits**
- **Caffeine**
  - An adenosine receptor antagonist, it can exert responses in many immune cells that have adenosine receptors
  - Ingestion results in elevated circulating epinephrine (adrenaline) allowing for indirect effects on immune cell functions through adrenoreceptor stimulation
  - Studies have shown increased lymphocyte responses following ingestion

Learn More: Sport Nutrition Textbook pgs 380-381

VITAMINS AND ANTIOXIDANTS AND IMMUNE FUNCTION

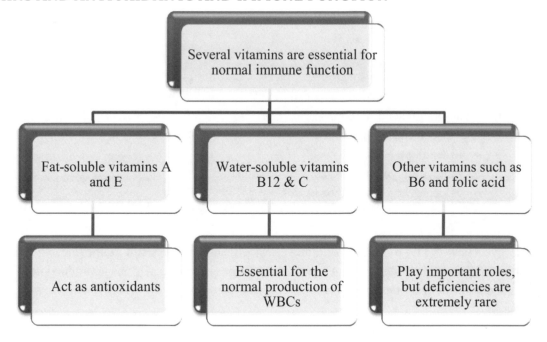

- Antioxidants including vitamins C, E and β-carotene may be required in increased quantities to deal with free-radical damage that can potentially inhibit immune responses

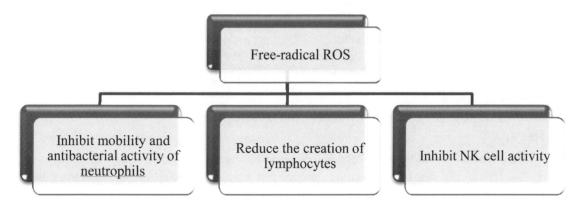

- Immunity-related antioxidant considerations:
  - Endurance training is associated with strengthening of the antioxidant defense system but innate protection may be insufficient during intense training, warranting extra intake
  - Mega-doses are not recommended as excess may blunt adaptations to training
  - Should be obtained through a variety of natural sources such as fruits and vegetables

Learn More: Sport Nutrition Textbook pgs 381-384

MINERALS AND IMMUNE FUNCTION

- Several minerals are essential for normal immune function, but deficiencies are rare with the exceptions of zinc and iron
- **Zinc**
    - o Essential for immune system development
    - o Facilitates enzyme reactions that result in immune cell replication
    - o Facilitates antioxidant functions
    - o Deficiency can cause:
        - ▪ Lymphoid atrophy
        - ▪ Impaired lymphocyte response to infection
        - ▪ Decreased cytokine production
        - ▪ Lowered NK cell activity
- **Iron**
    - o Necessary for O_2 transport; facilitates enzyme reactions that result in immune cell replication
    - o Deficiency depresses numerous immune functions such as macrophage production and lymphocyte reactions to infection
- **Selenium**
    - o Serves as an antioxidant cofactor
    - o Deficiency may allow for greater ROS-mediated cellular damage
- **Copper**
    - o Serves as an antioxidant cofactor
    - o Deficiency can:
        - ▪ Impair antibody formation
        - ▪ Reduce inflammatory responses
        - ▪ Impair neutrophil, NK cell, and lymphocyte activity
- **Magnesium and manganese**
    - o Inadequate intake can result in reduced antioxidant activity
- **Cobalt**
    - o Promotes the development of red and WBCs in bone marrow
    - o Deficiency can impair WBC count, lymphocyte reaction to infection, and bacteria-clearing capacity of neutrophils

Learn More: Sport Nutrition Textbook pgs 384-388

DIETARY IMMUNOSTIMULANTS

- **Echinacea**
    - o Several herbal preparations are reputed to be beneficial
    - o Macrophage activation has been demonstrated most convincingly
    - o An investigation involving 42 triathletes showed that daily oral ingestion of Echinacea purpurea juice for 28 days prior to sprint triathalon competition significantly reduced the incidence of illness post-competition when compared to magnesium or placebo
    - o Shown in research to provide modest benefits for treatment of acute URTI

- o True effectiveness in treating illness or enhancing health is still unclear
- **Probiotics**
  - o Function to increase the quantity of beneficial bacteria while reducing harmful bacteria
  - o May help inhibit growth and harmful effects of immodepressing bacteria, antigens, toxins, and carcinogens in the gut
  - o Directly interact with gut lymphoid tissue; 85% of the body's lymph nodes are located in the gut to deal with bacteria-mediated immunity challenges
  - o Studies have shown that probiotics
    - Improve the rate of recovery from rotavirus diarrhea
    - Provide increased resistance to intestinal pathogens
    - Promote antitumor activity
    - May help reduce stress-induced damage to the gut (i.e., GI disorders common among mountaineers due to altitude and exercise-induced stress)
    - May be effective in alleviating allergic and respiratory disorders in young children
- **Bovine Colostrum**
  - o Collection of a thick creamy yellow liquid produced by the mammary gland of a lactating cow shortly after giving birth, usually within 36 hours
  - o Contains:
    - Antibodies
    - Growth factors
    - Enzymes
    - Gangliosides (serve in cellular recognition and cell-to-cell communication)
      - May modify gut microbial flora, act as decoy targets for bacteria, and have direct immunostimulatory effects
    - Vitamins and minerals
  - o Health claims range from performance enhancement to preventing infections
  - o Well-controlled studies with athletes are rare; more research is needed to clarify if bovine colostrum can reduce the incidence of URTIs
- **β-Glucans**
  - o CHO-based structural components of the cell walls of yeast, fungi, some bacteria, and the endosperm cell wall in cereals such as barley and oats
  - o Effects depend on their characteristics and type
    - High-molecular-weight fungi directly activate WBCs
    - Low-molecular-weight fungi modify the response of immune cells only when stimulated by cytokines
  - o May be useful for specific populations - such as the elderly, type 2 diabetics, or athletes involved in heavy training - who may experience immune responses which β-glucans can alleviate
- *Other supplements*
  - o **Quercitin**
    - Type of flavonoid polyphenol
    - Shown in one study to significantly reduce URTI incidence in the 2 weeks following a short, intense training period

- o **Curcumin**
  - ▪ Orange-yellow component of turmeric, a spice often used in curry powder
  - ▪ Traditionally known for its anti-inflammatory effects
  - ▪ Shown in research to:
    - • Modify the activation of T-cells, B-cells, NK cells, neutrophils, macrophages, and dendritic cells (act as immunity messengers)
    - • Reduce expression of various pro-inflammatory cytokines

Learn More: Sport Nutrition Textbook pgs 389-392

PRACTICAL SUMMARY AND STRATEGIES TO MINIMIZE RISKS OF INFECTION

- Countering the effects of all the factors that contribute to exercise-induced immunodepression would be impossible, but optimizing the immune response is a reasonable goal
- Practical strategies to minimize the risk of infection during the competitive season
  - o Allow sufficient time between training sessions for recovery; include 1 or 2 days of rest in the weekly training program based on volume; more training is not always better
  - o Avoid extremely long training sessions; restrict activity to less than 2 hrs per session
  - o Avoid training monotony by ensuring variation in the day-to-day training load; follow a hard training day with less intense training day
  - o When increasing training load, do so on the hard days – do not eliminate recovery days
  - o When recovering from overtraining or illness, begin with very light training and build gradually
  - o Monitor and record mood, feelings of fatigue, and muscle soreness during training; decrease the training load if the normal training session feels harder than normal
  - o Keep other life, social, and psychological stresses to a minimum if possible
  - o Get regular and adequate sleep – at least 6 hrs/night
  - o Maintain good oral hygiene by brushing teeth regularly and using antiseptic mouthwash
  - o Wash hands regularly and do not share towels
  - o Increase rest as needed after travel across time zones to allow circadian rhythms to readjust
  - o Eat a well-balanced diet to obtain all the necessary vitamins and minerals
  - o If dieting to lose weight, or if fresh fruit and vegetables are not readily available, a multivitamin supplement may be useful
  - o Ensure adequate total dietary energy, CHO, and protein intake (be aware that periods of CHO depletion are associated with immunodepression)
  - o Drink CHO sports drinks before, during, and after prolonged training to reduce some of the adverse effects of exercise on immune function
  - o Consider discussing vaccination with a coach or doctor
    - ▪ Influenza vaccines require 5-7 weeks to take effect
    - ▪ Intramuscular vaccines may have a few small side effects; offseason vaccination is optimal
    - ▪ Never vaccinate before a competition or if symptoms of illness are present

Learn More: Sport Nutrition Textbook pgs 392-393

SECTION 3 • <u>REVIEW YOUR KNOWLEDGE</u>

<u>Match the Following Terms</u>

1. ____ Innate immunity   a. Innate immune system cell

2. ____ Echinacea   b. Deficiency can cause lymphoid atrophy

3. ____ NK cell   c. Activates lymphocyte actions to resist infection

4. ____ Adaptive immunity   d. Utilized at extremely high rates by WBCs

5. ____ Zinc   e. Consists of proteins that stimulate neutralization of infected cells

6. ____ Glutamine   f. First line of immune system defense

7. ____ Colostrum   g. Produced by a lactating cow shortly after birth

8. ____ Complement   h. May aid in the treatment of URTIs

<u>Knowledge and Competency Exercises</u>

11. Describe three actions that occur during the inflammatory response.

a) _____

b) _____

c) _____

12. Macrophages first _____ invading microorganisms to metabolize proteins on its surface, and then activate _____ and _____ specific for eradicating the infectious agent.

13. List four practices that can minimize the risk of infection during the early recovery period after exercise.

a) _____

b) _____

c) _____

d) _____

14. True or False? *(circle one)* Circulating WBC counts are generally lower in athletes at rest when compared with sedentary individuals.

15. List five immune system functions that can be compromised with low nutrient availability.

a) _____   b) _____   c) _____

d) _____   e) _____

16. Exercising in a CHO-depleted state can cause larger increases in circulating _____, reduced _____ availability, and _____ effects on immune functions.

17. True or False? *(circle one)* Fatty acids can exert effects on the immune system by altering cell membrane fluidity and reducing eicosanoid formation.

18. True or False? *(circle one)* Studies show increased lymphocyte activity within the body following the ingestion of caffeine.

19. List three negative effects related to immune function caused by free radical ROS.

a) _____

b) _____

c) _____

20. _____ promotes the development of red and WBCs in bone marrow.

21. True or False? *(circle one)* Echinacea has been shown in research to provide modest benefits for treatment of acute URTIs.

22. Describe five practical strategies that athletes should consider to minimize the risk of infection during the competitive season.

a) _____

b) _____

c) _____

d) _____

e) _____

• ASSESS YOUR KNOWLEDGE

SECTION 4

1. Which of the following is <u>not</u> a component of innate immunity?

   a. Skin
   b. Chemical barriers
   c. Phagocytes
   d. Lymphocytes

2. Which of the following changes related to immune function occur during the recovery period after exercise which can increase the risk of infection?

   a. An increase in circulating WBCs
   b. A decrease in cortisol production
   c. An increase in plasma glutamine concentration
   d. NK cell numbers and activity fall below pre-exercise levels

3. Consuming _____ during exercise reduces stress hormones and appears to limit the degree of exercise-induced immunodepression.

   a. Glutamine
   b. PUFAs
   c. CHOs
   d. Echinacea

4. Inadequate protein intake can negatively impair the immune system in which of the following ways?

   a. Enhanced T-cell lymphocyte activity
   b. Widespread atrophy of lymphoid tissue
   c. Enhanced phagocytic immune cell activity
   d. Increased cytokine production and activity

5. Evidence suggests that consumption of light to moderate amounts of _____ alcoholic beverages such as wine could have health benefits.

   a. Polyphenol-rich
   b. CHO-rich
   c. PUFA-rich
   d. Probiotic-rich

6. Deficiency of _____ can cause lymphoid atrophy, impaired lymphocyte responses to infection, decreased cytokine production, and lowered NK cell activity.

    a. Zinc
    b. Iron
    c. Copper
    d. Cobalt

7. Which of the following dietary immunostimulants is derived from the mammary gland of a lactating cow shortly after giving birth?

    a. Echinacea
    b. β-glucans
    c. Bovine colostrum
    d. Curcumin

8. Of the following statements concerning probiotics, which is <u>INCORRECT</u>?

    a. They can directly interact with 85% of the body's lymph nodes
    b. They may be effective in alleviating some allergic reactions and respiratory disorders in young children
    c. They can help inhibit the growth and harmful effects of immunodepressing bacteria, toxins, and carcinogens in the gut
    d. They can improve the rate of recovery from viral influenza

9. Which of the following is a vitamin considered to be essential for normal immune function?

    a. Selenium
    b. Vitamin B_{12}
    c. Vitamin K
    d. Iron

10. Vaccinations are optimally attained during _____ and never before _____.

    a. The in-season, sleeping
    b. The off-season, competition
    c. The pre-season, eating
    d. Competition, the off-season

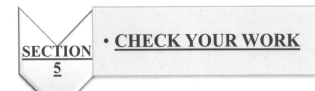

• CHECK YOUR WORK

SPORT NUTRITION CHAPTER 16 ANSWERS

Match the Following Terms

1. F

2. H

3. A

4. C

5. B

6. D

7. G

8. E

Knowledge and Competency Exercises

11. **a)** Increased local blood flow to the infected area, **b)** Increased permeability of local capillaries, **c)** Allows entry of WBCs and plasma proteins into the infected tissue

12. Ingest, lymphocytes, antibodies

13. **Possible answers**: Avoid contact with people who have symptoms of infection, minimize contact with school-age children and large crowds, wash hands regularly, particularly after touching surfaces frequently handled by the public, avoid hand-to-eye and hand-to-mouth contact to prevent transferring microbes to sensitive mucosal tissues, maintain good oral hygiene, avoid getting a dry mouth during competition and at rest by drinking at regular intervals and maintaining hydration status, never share drink bottles or cutlery, use properly treated water for consumption and swimming, avoid shared saunas, showers, and whirlpool tubs

14. True

15. **a)** Antibody production, **b)** inter-cellular immunity, **c)** capacity of phagocytes to kill bacteria, **d)** complement formation, **e)** lymphocyte creation

16. Stress hormones, glutamine, greater negative

17. False

18. True

19. **a)** Inhibited mobility and bactericidal activity of neutrophils, **b)** Reduced creation of lymphocytes, **c)** Inhibited NK cell activity

20. Cobalt

21. True

22. **Possible answers:** Allow sufficient time between training sessions for recovery, avoid extremely long training sessions, avoid training monotony by ensuring variation in the day-to-day training load, when increasing training load, do so on the hard days, when recovering from overtraining or illness, begin with very light training and build gradually, monitor and record mood, feelings of fatigue, and muscle soreness during training, keep other life, social, and psychological stresses to a minimum, get at least 6 hours of sleep each night, maintain good oral hygiene by brushing teeth regularly and using antiseptic mouthwash, wash hands regularly and do not share towels, increase rest as needed after travel across time zones to allow circadian rhythms to adjust, eat a well-balanced diet to obtain all the necessary vitamins and minerals, if dieting to lose weight or if fresh fruit and vegetables are not readily available - use a multivitamin supplement, ensure adequate total dietary energy, CHO, and protein intake, drink CHO sports drinks before, during, and after prolonged training, consider discussing vaccination with a coach or doctor

Assess Your Knowledge

1. D

2. D

3. C

4. B

5. A

6. A

7. C

8. D

9. B

10. B